Drugs in Obstetrics, Gynecology, and Reproductive Endocrinology

Drugs in Obstetrics, Gynecology, and Reproductive Endocrinology

Editor
Pratik Tambe
MD FICOG
ART Consultant and Gynec Endoscopic Surgeon
Ashirwad IVF
Mumbai, Maharashtra, India
Governing Council Member, ICOG (2020–25)
Chairperson, AMOGS Endocrinology Committee (2020–24)
Managing Council Member, MOGS, ISAR, MSR
Chairperson, FOGSI Endocrinology Committee (2017–19)

Foreword
Nandita Palshetkar

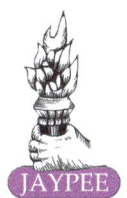

JAYPEE BROTHERS MEDICAL PUBLISHERS
The Health Sciences Publisher
New Delhi | London

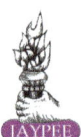 Jaypee Brothers Medical Publishers (P) Ltd

Headquarters

Jaypee Brothers Medical Publishers (P) Ltd
EMCA House, 23/23-B
Ansari Road, Daryaganj
New Delhi 110 002, India
Landline: +91-11-23272143, +91-11-23272703
+91-11-23282021, +91-11-23245672
Email: jaypee@jaypeebrothers.com

Corporate Office

Jaypee Brothers Medical Publishers (P) Ltd
4838/24, Ansari Road, Daryaganj
New Delhi 110 002, India
Phone: +91-11-43574357
Fax: +91-11-43574314
Email: jaypee@jaypeebrothers.com

Overseas Office

JP Medical Ltd
83 Victoria Street, London
SW1H 0HW (UK)
Phone: +44 20 3170 8910
Fax: +44 (0)20 3008 6180
Email: info@jpmedpub.com

Website: www.jaypeebrothers.com
Website: www.jaypeedigital.com

© 2024, Jaypee Brothers Medical Publishers

The views and opinions expressed in this book are solely those of the original contributor(s)/author(s) and do not necessarily represent those of editor(s) or publisher of the book.

All rights reserved. No part of this publication may be reproduced, stored or transmitted in any form or by any means, electronic, mechanical, photocopying, recording or otherwise, without the prior permission in writing of the publishers.

All brand names and product names used in this book are trade names, service marks, trademarks or registered trademarks of their respective owners. The publisher is not associated with any product or vendor mentioned in this book.

Medical knowledge and practice change constantly. This book is designed to provide accurate, authoritative information about the subject matter in question. However, readers are advised to check the most current information available on procedures included and check information from the manufacturer of each product to be administered, to verify the recommended dose, formula, method and duration of administration, adverse effects and contraindications. It is the responsibility of the practitioner to take all appropriate safety precautions. Neither the publisher nor the author(s)/editor(s) assume any liability for any injury and/or damage to persons or property arising from or related to use of material in this book.

This book is sold on the understanding that the publisher is not engaged in providing professional medical services. If such advice or services are required, the services of a competent medical professional should be sought.

Every effort has been made where necessary to contact holders of copyright to obtain permission to reproduce copyright material. If any have been inadvertently overlooked, the publisher will be pleased to make the necessary arrangements at the first opportunity.

Inquiries for bulk sales may be solicited at: jaypee@jaypeebrothers.com

Drugs in Obstetrics, Gynecology, and Reproductive Endocrinology

First Edition: **2024**

ISBN: 978-93-5696-549-2

Contributors

Ameya Purandare MD DNB FCPS DGO DFP MNAMS FICMCH FICOG Fellowship in Gyne Endoscopy (Germany)
Senior Consultant Obstetrician and Gynecologist
Purandare Hospital, KJ Somaiya Medical College and Hospital
Sir HN Reliance Foundation Hospital and Research Centre
Bhatia Hospital, Masina Hospital
Mumbai Police Hospital
Mumbai, Maharashtra, India
Vice President, Association of Maharashtra Obstetrics and Gynaecological Societies (AMOGS) (2022–2024)
Joint Secretary, FOGSI, 2019
Chairperson, Food, Drugs and Medical and Surgical Equipment Committee, FOGSI (2015–2017)
Assistant Administrator, FOGSI Manyata Project

Anjali Suneel Mundkur
MS DNB MRCOG
Associate Professor
Department of Reproductive Medicine and Surgery
Kasturba Medical College
Manipal, Karnataka, India

Basab Mukherjee MD FRCOG FICOG
Consultant
Department of Obstetrics and Gynecology
Woodlands Multispecialty Hospital
Kolkata, West Bengal, India
Past Vice President, FOGSI
President, Bengal Obs/Gyn Society
Past Chairperson
FOGSI Family Welfare Committee

Bhaskar Pal
MD DGO DNBE MRCOG FICOG FRCOG
Senior Consultant
Department of Obstetrics and Gynecology
Apollo Multispeciality Hospital
Kolkata, West Bengal, India
Chair AICC RCOG
FOGSI Representative to SAFOG
Immediate Past President, IAGE
Co-Chair, Endoscopy Committee SAFOG
Past Vice President, FOGSI
Past President, Bengal Obs/Gyn Society
Past Chair, AICC RCOG East Zone
Past Chair, FOGSI Young Talent Promotion Committee

Charmila Ayyavoo
MD DGO DFP FICOG PGDCR
Director
Department of Obstetrics and Gynecology
Aditi Hospital, Southern Railway Hospital
Tiruchirappalli, Tamil Nadu, India
Vice President Elect, FOGSI
Past Chairperson
FOGSI Clinical Research Committee

Krishnendu Gupta MBBS DGO MD FICMCH FICOG FRCPI FRCOG (Ad Eundem, UK) FACOG (Hon, USA)
Professor and Unit Head
Department of Obstetrics and Gynecology
Vivekananda Institute of Medical Sciences
Kolkata, West Bengal, India
Past Vice President, FOGSI
Deputy Secretary General, AOFOG

Kuldeep Jain MD Fellowship ART
Director
Department of Reproductive Medicine
KJIVF and Laparoscopy Center
New Delhi, India
Past President
Indian Fertility Society
Past Chairperson
FOGSI Endometriosis Committee

Maansi Jain MS Fellowship ART
Consultant
Department of Reproductive Medicine
KJIVF and Laparoscopy Center
New Delhi, India

Manisha Nandi MBBS MS (Obs/Gyne)
FRM (Fellowship in Reproductive Medicine)
DRME (Germany)
Fellow Reproductive Medicine (IVF)
DY Patil Medical College
Kolkata, West Bengal, India

N Sanjeeva Reddy MD (Obs/Gyne)
Professor
Department of Reproductive Medicine
and Surgery
Sri Ramachandra Institute of Higher
Education and Research
Chennai, Tamil Nadu, India
Chairperson, Tamil Nadu and
Pondicherry Chapter, ISAR

Nandita Palshetkar
MD DGO FCPS FICOG FRCOG
Medical Director, Bloom IVF-India
Mumbai, Maharashtra, India
President, ISAR (2022–24)
Past President, FOGSI, IAGE, AMOGS, MOGS
FOGSI Representative to FIGO

Neharika Malhotra MD (Obs/Gyne)
(Gold Medalist) DRM (Germany) FICOG
Infertility Consultant
Rainbow IVF
Agra, Uttar Pradesh, India
Chairperson, FOGSI Young Talent
Promotion Committee

Parag Biniwale MD
Chief Consultant and Director
Department of Obstetrics and
Gynecology
Biniwale Clinic
Pune, Maharashtra, India
Vice Chair, ICOG
Past President
Pune Obs/Gyn Society

Parikshit Tank MD DNB FCPS DGO DFP
MNAMS FICOG FRCOG
Consultant
Department of Obstetrics and Gynecology
Ashwini Maternity and Surgical Hospital
Center for Endoscopy and Assisted
Reproduction
Mumbai, Maharashtra, India
Treasurer, FOGSI
Joint Clinical Secretary, MOGS

PK Shah MD FCPS DGO DFP
Professor and Head of Unit
Department of Obstetrics and
Gynecology
Geetanjali Medical College and Hospital
Udaipur, Rajasthan, India
Past President FOGSI, IAGE, MOGS, IFUMB

Poushali Sanyal
MS DNB MRCOG FMAS FICOG
Consultant
Department of Obstetrics and
Gynecology
Woodlands Multispecialty Hospital
Kolkata, West Bengal, India

Pratap Kumar Narayan MD FICOG FICS
Professor and Head
Department of Reproductive Medicine
and Surgery
Kasturba Medical College
Manipal, Karnataka, India
Past Vice President, FOGSI

Contributors

Pratik Tambe MD FICOG
ART Consultant and Gynec Endoscopic Surgeon
Ashirwad IVF
Mumbai, Maharashtra, India
Governing Council Member, ICOG (2020–25)
Chairperson, AMOGS Endocrinology Committee (2020–24)
Managing Council Member, MOGS, ISAR, MSR
Chairperson, FOGSI Endocrinology Committee (2017–19)

Radha Vembu
MBBS DGO DNB PhD MNAMS FICS FICOG
Professor and Head
Department of Reproductive Medicine and Surgery
Sri Ramachandra Medical College and Research Institute
Chennai, Tamil Nadu, India

Riddhi Desai MS FICOG PGDMLS
Dip Endoscopy (Pune, USA) Dip Office Hysteroscopy (Italy)
Senior Consultant, Sunflower Clinics
Mumbai, Maharashtra, India
Managing Council Member, MOGS
Member, Youth Brigade PCOS Society of India

Rohan Palshetkar MS (Obs/Gyne) FRM
Head of Unit, DY Patil Bloom IVF
Associate Professor
DY Patil School of Medicine
Consultant Obstetrics and Gynecology
Sir HN Reliance Foundation Hospital, Surya Hospital, Breach Candy Hospital, DY Patil Hospital, Palshetkar Patil Nursing Home
Mumbai, Maharashtra, India
Treasurer, AMOGS
Joint Treasurer, Maharashtra Chapter of IAGE
Managing Committee Member of Mumbai Obstetrics and Gynaecological Society and Maharashtra Chapter of ISAR

Samidha Dalvi MBBS DNB (Obs/Gyne)
Fellowship in Infertility (Spain)
Medical Director and Clinical Head
Department of Reproductive Medicine
Pune IVF Fertility Centre and Research Institute
Pune, Maharashtra, India

Seema Pandey
MBBS MS FICOG FRM
Director and Consultant
Department of Reproductive Medicine
Seema Hospital and Eva Fertility Clinic and IVF Center
Azamgarh, Uttar Pradesh, India
Managing Committee Member, ISAR

Suchitra Pandit
MD DNB FRCOG DFP FICOG BPharm
Consultant Obstetrics and Gynecology
Surya Group of Hospitals, Mumbai
Former Consultant and Head
Kokilaben Dhirubhai Ambani Hospital
Mumbai, Maharashtra, India
President, Gestosis India Association
Chair, AICC RCOG (2017–20)
President ISOPARB (2018–20)
Chairperson, Medical Education SAFOG (2017–2019)
President, FOGSI and ICOG (2014–15)
President, MOGS (2013–14)
Vice Chair, ICOG (2010-2011)

Sujoy Dasgupta
MS DNB MRCOG MSc
Consultant and Clinical Director
Department of Reproductive Medicine
Genome Fertility Centre
Kolkata, West Bengal, India

Umme Ruman
MBBS (Gold Medal) FCPS (Obs/Gyne)
Infertility and IVF Specialist
Associate Professor
East West Medical College
Dhaka, Bangladesh

Foreword

I am extremely pleased to pen down the foreword to the book on *Drugs in Obstetrics, Gynecology, and Reproductive Endocrinology*.

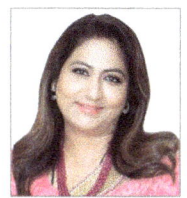

The world of medicine is constantly evolving, and new treatments are being developed every day. Newer drug treatments for gynecological conditions and in the field of reproductive endocrinology are now available compared to 1–2 decades ago. With the rise of new technologies and a deeper understanding of the human body, researchers are discovering new ways to treat and manage diseases. In many clinical conditions, these newer molecules have revolutionized therapeutic approaches and created a wider array of choices available to both clinicians and patients.

This book focuses on some of the most happening molecules and the current evidence for the same. The chapters have been authored by senior clinicians across the length and breadth of the country who have brought their experience and expertise to the table while writing about these formulations.

In addition to discussing these latest treatments, the authors have also delved into the science behind these drugs and therapies. They extensively discuss the mechanisms of action of the drugs and how they interact with the body to produce their effects. Due importance is also given to the potential side effects and risks associated with these treatments, as well as their benefits and limitations.

I hope this focused volume will go a long way toward being an easy guide and quick reference to the newer approaches that we should today offer our patients in the light of good clinical evidence which is now available. My hearty congratulations to the Editor, Dr Pratik Tambe and all the contributors for their hard work and effort which will surely benefit the readers of this book.

Nandita Palshetkar
MD DGO FCPS FICOG FRCOG
Medical Director, Bloom IVF-India
President, ISAR (2022–24)
Past President, FOGSI, IAGE, AMOGS, MOGS
FOGSI Representative to FIGO

Preface

Ars longa, vita brevis – Hippocrates

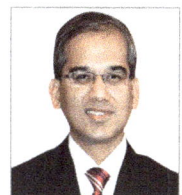

The field of medicine has always been in a state of constant evolution, with new drugs and treatment methodologies being developed and tested every year. As healthcare professionals, it is our responsibility to stay updated with the latest advancements in medicine to ensure that our patients receive the best possible care. In this textbook, we aim to provide a comprehensive overview of the latest drugs and treatment methodologies that have emerged in recent years.

The pharmaceutical industry has made tremendous strides in developing new drugs that target-specific diseases and conditions. In this book, we will explore some of the most promising new drugs that have been developed recently. These drugs are designed to be more effective and have fewer side effects than traditional medications. We will examine the mechanisms of action for each drug, as well as their clinical applications and potential side effects.

Finally, we recognize that the field of medicine is constantly evolving, and new drugs and treatment methodologies are being introduced all the time. Therefore, this book is intended to be a living document that will be updated regularly to reflect the latest advancements in medicine. We encourage readers to provide feedback and suggestions for future editions so that we can continue to provide the most up-to-date information possible.

In conclusion, we believe that this textbook will be a valuable resource for healthcare professionals who are looking to stay informed about the latest developments in medicine. I hope that readers will find this book informative and engaging and I look forward to continuing this important conversation as the field of medicine continues to evolve.

I thank all the esteemed authors and co-authors for the timely submission of the chapters. I am highly indebted to Dr Nandita Palshetkar, President, ISAR, for her blessings and support for all my academic endeavors over the years. I would also like to express my gratitude to the publishers—M/s Jaypee Brothers Medical Publishers (P) Ltd, Ms Chetna Malhotra (Senior Director—Professional Publishing, Marketing, and Business Development), Kritika Dua (Senior Development Editor), and Pragati Singh (Development Editor), for their hard work and coordination to enable the timely release of this volume.

Pratik Tambe
Editor

Contents

1. **Carbetocin** 1
   Pratik Tambe, Parikshit Tank
   Postpartum Hemorrhage *1*;   World Health Organization Recommendations *1*;   Scientific Evidence *3*;   Guideline Recommendations *3*;   Recent Evidence *4*;   Cost-Effectiveness and Hurdles to Implementation *5*

2. **Ulipristal Acetate** 7
   Charmila Ayyavoo
   Mode of Action *7*;   Uses *8*;   Side Effects *9*;   Dosages Advised *10*

3. **Dydrogesterone** 13
   Bhaskar Pal, Poushali Sanyal, Sujoy Dasgupta
   Pharmacology *13*;   Immunomodulation *13*;   Luteal Phase Support in Assisted Reproductive Technology *14*;   Suppression of Luteinizing Hormone in Assisted Reproductive Technology *15*;   Threatened Miscarriage *16*;   Recurrent Miscarriage *16*;   Emerging Applications *17*;   Safety Concerns *17*

4. **Dehydroepiandrosterone (DHEA)** 21
   Nandita Palshetkar, Pratik Tambe
   In vitro Fertilization *21*;   Role of Dehydroepiandrosterone in Fertility *22*;   Mechanisms of Action *22*;   Altered Gene Expression *22*;   Cellular Apoptosis *23*;   Mitochondrial Function *23*;   Senescence and Aging *23*;   Dosage and Treatment Duration *24*;   Clinical Evidence *24*;   Largest Meta-analysis and Systematic Review *25*;   Controversies to Consensus *25*;   Directions for Future Research *26*

5. **Dienogest** 29
   Kuldeep Jain, Maansi Jain
   Chemical Structure *29*;   Mechanism of Action *29*;   Side Effects *30*;   Dosage and Efficacy *30*

6. ***Lactobacillus* spp.** 33
   Pratap Kumar Narayan, Anjali Suneel Mundkur
   Types *33*;   Lactobacilli in Gastrointestinal Tract *34*;   *Lactobacillus* in the Female Genital Tract *35*;   Lactobacilli as Vaginal Probiotic *36*;   Clinical Uses of Probiotics *37*;   Uses of Probiotics in Restoring Reproductive Health in Women *38*;   Safety and Side Effects of Probiotics *38*

7. **Melatonin** 41
   Suchitra Pandit, Pratik Tambe
   Overview of Melatonin *41*;   Lifestyle Factors and Oxidative Stress *43*;   Melatonin and the Testis *43*;   Scientific Evidence *44*;   Clinical Application *44*;   Melatonin and Assisted Reproductive Techniques Outcomes *45*;   Ovarian Antiaging *45*

8. **New Generation Oral Contraceptive Pills**..49
   Neharika Malhotra, Umme Ruman
   Aim 49; Discussion 49; Change in Components 50;
   Categories of Pill 50; Newer Combined Oral Contraceptive Pill 52;
   Newer Progesterone-Only Pill 53

9. **Parenteral Iron** 57
   PK Shah
   Stages of Iron Deficiency 57; Oral Iron Therapy 57; Intravenous Iron 58;
   Intramuscular Iron Preparations 60; Hypersensitivity Reactions 60

10. **Berberine**..65
    Pratik Tambe
    History 65; Mechanism of Action 65; Insulin Resistance 66;
    Androgen Levels 67; Dosage 67; Health Benefits and Clinical
    Applications 67; Scientific Evidence for Combination Therapy 69

11. **Astaxanthin** 75
    Parag Biniwale, Samidha Dalvi
    Source of Astaxanthin 75; Structure of Astaxanthin 75; Biochemistry of
    Astaxanthin 75; Bioavailability and Pharmacokinetics of Astaxanthin 77;
    Biological Activities of Astaxanthin and its Health Benefits 77; Safety and
    Dose of Astaxanthin 78; Astraxanthin in Infertility 78; Astaxanthin in
    Obstetrics 80

12. **Levonorgestrel Intrauterine System** 81
    Krishnendu Gupta, Pratik Tambe
    Device Characteristics 81; Mechanism of Action 82; Device Insertion 82;
    Contraceptive Benefits 82; Utility in Heavy Menstrual Bleeding 83;
    Endometriosis-associated Pelvic Pain 86; Side Effects 86

13. **Coenzyme Q10** 91
    N Sanjeeva Reddy, Radha Vembu
    Female Infertility 91; Male Infertility 94

14. **Quatrefolate: The Fourth-Generation Folate**............................101
    Ameya Purandare, Rohan Palshetkar, Manisha Nandi
    Folic Acid and 5-Methyltetrahydrofolate 101; Health Benefits of the
    Drug 102; Pharmacokinetics 106; Chemical Stability (At Room
    Temperature) 106; Toxicological Studies 107; Recent Updates:
    The Active Folate and Pregnancy Outcome Versus Folic Acid 108

15. **Gonadotropins in Prefilled Syringe Form** 111
    Seema Pandey, Pratik Tambe
    Prefilled Syringe Concept 111; Comparison with Traditional
    Formulations 111; Usage in Other Specialties of Medicine 114;
    Scientific Evidence 114; Disadvantages 114

16. **Etonogestrel Implant**..117
    Basab Mukherjee, Riddhi Desai
    Etonogestrel 117; Etonogestrel Implant 118; Training and Expertise 120;
    Cost-effectiveness in India 121

Index 123

CHAPTER 1

Carbetocin

Pratik Tambe, Parikshit Tank

■ BACKGROUND

Postpartum hemorrhage (PPH) is one of the most important causes of maternal morbidity and mortality in current clinical practice. Blood loss of >500 mL at vaginal delivery (VD) or 1,000 mL at cesarean section is considered significant. It accounts for 13% maternal deaths in the Western world and 28% of maternal deaths in developing countries.[1]

While the maternal mortality has declined significantly in India over the past few decades, much needs to be done to bring it in line with western standards. In India, the maternal mortality rate (MMR) declined by about 70% from 398/100,000 live births [95% confidence interval (CI) 378–417] in 1997–1998 to 99/100,000 (90–108) in 2020. The MMRs for Assam (215), Uttar Pradesh/Uttarakhand (192), and Madhya Pradesh/Chhattisgarh (170) were highest, surpassing India's 2016–2018 estimate of 113 (95% CI 103–123). The leading causes of maternal death were obstetric hemorrhage (47%), pregnancy-related infection (12%), and hypertensive disorders of pregnancy (7%).[2]

■ POSTPARTUM HEMORRHAGE

Postpartum hemorrhage may lead to sequelae such as massive blood transfusion, intensive care unit (ICU) admission, and even obstetric hysterectomy. It is unpredictable as it occurs without identifiable clinical or historical risk factors. Hence, effective prevention strategies such as the active management of the third stage of labor (AMTSL) are advocated in routine clinical practice. Great emphasis is placed upon the use of a prophylactic uterotonic drug as it reduces the risk of PPH by 66%.[3]

■ WORLD HEALTH ORGANIZATION RECOMMENDATIONS

Among the uterotonics available include oxytocin, ergometrine, and misoprostol, carbetocin is a newer option. The World Health Organization (WHO) previously recommended one dose of oxytocin (10 IU) as the drug of choice for the prevention of PPH. The WHO has also recently considered

2 Carbetocin

carbetocin as a prophylactic uterotonic of choice, if carbetocin were a cost-effective choice.[4]

Carbetocin is a synthetic analog of oxytocin and functions as an alternative to oxytocin (**Figs. 1 and 2**). It has a longer half-life of 41 minutes, allowing it to stimulate a prolonged uterine response of up to an hour after a single intravenous (IV) dose, obviating the need for infusion.

However, its greatest advantage is that it is heat-stable and can be stored at room temperature. It has been proven to retain its efficacy when stored

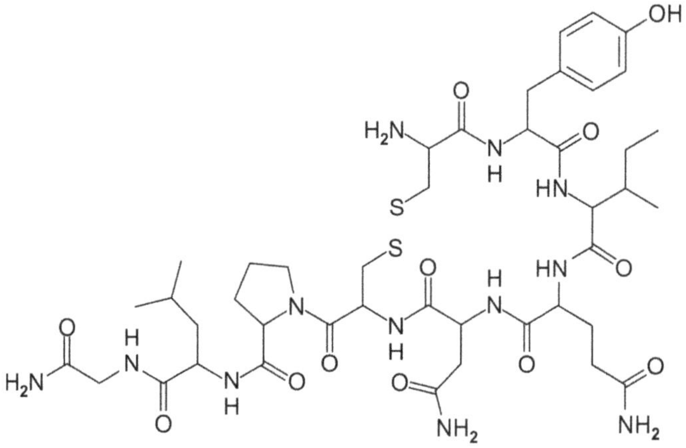

Fig. 1: Chemical structure of oxytocin.

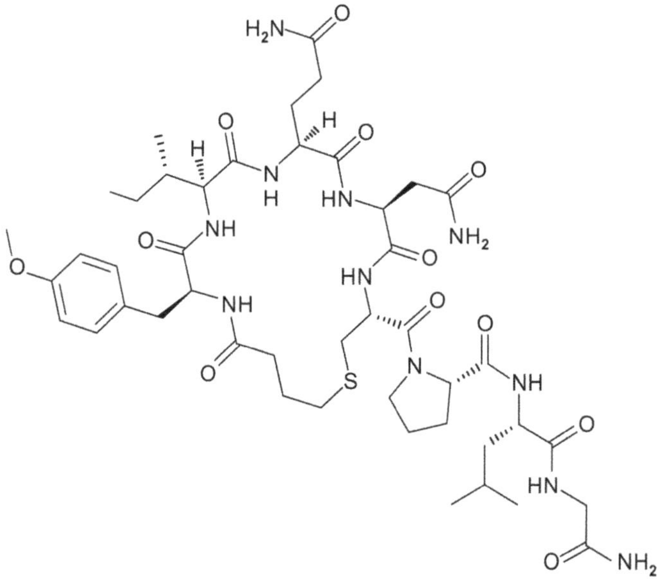

Fig. 2: Chemical structure of carbetocin.

at 30°C for 36 months, which is appealing in a country like India where cold chain maintenance is a challenge, especially in the interiors and states where maternal mortality is high and infrastructure is poor.

A Cochrane meta-analysis published in 2018 by Gallos et al. illustrated a longer duration of action compared with oxytocin, reducing the need for additional doses [relative risk (RR) 0.48, 95% CI 0.34–0.68]. It was clinically effective in PPH prevention in VD (PPH ≥500 mL 0.67, 95% CI 0.34–1.30) and in CS (PPH ≥1,000 mL 0.62, 95% CI 0.31–1.23) with comparable side effect profile to oxytocin.[1,5]

■ SCIENTIFIC EVIDENCE

A systematic review by Lawrie et al. reviewed the cost-effectiveness of uterotonics, including carbetocin and oxytocin and included 15 economic evaluations. Multiple databases were searched and articles published until 2018 were retrieved. The Cochrane meta-analysis by Gallos et al. included 140 randomized controlled trials (RCTs) available published until October 2017, to conduct a network meta-analysis of uterotonics.[1,6]

In the comparison network for the outcome of PPH ≥500 mL and ≥1,000 mL, eight and seven studies directly compared carbetocin with oxytocin, respectively. Voon et al. searched multiple databases and included seven RCTs published until May 2016. 22 major publications including guidelines and meta-analyses were included in a Canadian Journal of Health Technologies Rapid Response Report published 2019.[7]

There is evidence to support the use of carbetocin for the prevention of PPH of ≥500 mL or ≥1,000 mL based on a network meta-analysis. In a subgroup analysis and a smaller systematic review, carbetocin was more effective than oxytocin for PPH prevention for cesarean delivery and not VD. In the primary studies, carbetocin was associated with similar or greater effectiveness regarding the prevention of PPH, reducing additional uterotonic use or hemoglobin drops.

In the systematic review of economic evaluations, carbetocin was more cost-effective than oxytocin for the prevention of PPH. From a UK perspective, carbetocin, oxytocin, and another uterotonic agents were considered the most cost-effective strategies for preventing PPH.

■ GUIDELINE RECOMMENDATIONS

According to a 2018 Canadian guideline, carbetocin is recommended to prevent PPH for cesarean delivery and VD with one PPH risk factor. Carbetocin is also considered first-line treatment in a 2018 German guideline.

Carbetocin 100 μg given as an IV bolus over 1 minute should be used instead of continuous oxytocin infusion in elective cesarean section for the prevention of PPH and to decrease the need for therapeutic uterotonics (Grade 1-B).

For women delivering vaginally with one risk factor for PPH, carbetocin 100 µg intramuscular (IM) decreases the need for uterine massage to prevent PPH when compared with continuous infusion of oxytocin (Grade 1-B).[8]

As per the Royal College of Obstetricians and Gynaecologists (RCOG) guideline, carbetocin is licensed in the UK specifically for the indication of prevention of PPH in the context of cesarean delivery. Use of carbetocin resulted in a statistically significant reduction in the need for further uterotonics compared with oxytocin for those undergoing a cesarean, but not for VD.

Available research does not clearly support the use of one particular uterotonic over another for second-line treatment of primary PPH due to uterine atony (ergot alkaloids, prostaglandins, and carbetocin). Midwives should choose their second-line uterotonic based on clinical context (strong recommendation; very low quality evidence).[9]

■ RECENT EVIDENCE

A meta-analysis of five RCTs (30,314 women) comparing carbetocin and oxytocin concluded that there was no significant difference between the two as regards blood loss ≥500 mL during VD (RR 0.52; 95% CI 0.24–1.15; $p = 0.11$; $I_2 = 69\%$). No significant differences were found in blood loss ≥1,000 mL, use of additional uterotonic agents, blood transfusion, uterine massage, flushing, vomiting, abdominal pain, nausea, dizziness, headache, palpitation, itching, and shivering.[10]

A systematic review and meta-analysis conducted in 2022 of three RCTs with 404 patients comparing IV carbetocin and rectal misoprostol concluded that the former was a superior substitute to the latter for active management of the third stage of labor.

The IV carbetocin group had significantly lower blood loss, need for additional uterotonics, uterine massage, and blood transfusion compared to the rectal misoprostol group. As regards the adverse effects, the rates of diarrhea and chills were significantly lower in the IV carbetocin group compared to the rectal misoprostol group.[11]

CHAMPION Trial

A total of 23 sites in 10 countries had 29,645 women enrolled in a randomized, double-blind, noninferiority trial comparing IM heat stable carbetocin (100 µg) versus oxytocin (10 IU) after vaginal birth.

The frequency of blood loss of at least 500 mL or the use of additional uterotonic agents was 14.5% in the carbetocin group and 14.4% in the oxytocin group (RR 1.01; 95% CI 0.95–1.06), a finding that was consistent with noninferiority. The use of additional uterotonic agents, interventions to stop bleeding, and adverse effects did not differ significantly between the two groups.

The trial concluded that heat stable carbetocin was noninferior to oxytocin for the prevention of blood loss of at least 500 mL or the use of additional uterotonic agents. Seven sites out of 23 were from India, which makes the CHAMPION trial particularly relevant to obstetric practices in India.[12]

COST-EFFECTIVENESS AND HURDLES TO IMPLEMENTATION

A systematic review indicated that seven out of eight cost-effectiveness studies involving carbetocin and oxytocin in high-, upper-middle, or middle-income countries concluded that carbetocin was cost-effective for CS, but no similar studies in low- and middle-income countries (LMICs) were identified.

An economic evaluation whether carbetocin would represent good value for money in an LMIC like the Philippines was recently published. The authors noted that the price of carbetocin (13.10–25.60 USD) is significantly more expensive compared with oxytocin (0.27 USD). They concluded that carbetocin is not a cost-effective choice in PPH prevention for both modes of delivery in the Philippines, unless a price reduction is made.[5]

A more recent scoping review on implementation of heat stable carbetocin concluded that there is a lack of evidence on the feasibility beyond cost-effectiveness, acceptability, and health system considerations related to implementation in resource-constrained and lower level maternity facilities. Further implementation research is needed to help decision makers and practitioners offer an intervention package to prevent excessive bleeding among pregnant women living in settings where oxytocin is not available or of dubious quality.[13]

Similarly, no such comparative study is available for India but pricing is quite similar. After a short interval, the maximum retail price (MRP) of the drug will probably be lower once it is widely embraced throughout the country and economies of scale kick in.

CONCLUSION

Carbetocin in its heat stable form can be preserved at room temperature of 30°C for 36 months and in a country like India where cold chain maintenance is a major issue, this in conjunction with its longer half-life will prove to be a boon in reducing maternal mortality owing to PH.

There is ample evidence demonstrating carbetocin is similarly or more effective than oxytocin for the prevention of PPH, especially for cesarean section deliveries. It is now recommended by the WHO and international guidelines from various authorities including the RCOG and the Canadian Society. Currently, it is considered more cost-effective than oxytocin in certain studies. Though the prevailing pricing is higher than oxytocin, it is expected that over time the MRP will be lower once it is more widely adopted as the agent of choice in the prevention of PPH.

REFERENCES

1. Gallos ID, Williams HM, Price MJ, Merriel A, Gee H, Lissauer D, et al. Uterotonic agents for preventing postpartum haemorrhage: a network meta-analysis. Cochrane Database Syst Rev. 2018;4:CD011689.
2. Meh C, Sharma A, Ram U, Fadel S, Correa N, Snelgrove JW, et al. Trends in maternal mortality in India over two decades in nationally representative surveys. BJOG. 2021;129(4):550-61.
3. van der Nelson HA, Draycott T, Siassakos D, Yau CWH, Hatswell AJ. Carbetocin versus oxytocin for prevention of post-partum haemorrhage at caesarean section in the United Kingdom: an economic impact analysis. Eur J Obstet Gynecol Reprod Biol. 2017;210:286-91.
4. World Health Organization. WHO recommendations for the prevention and treatment of postpartum haemorrhage. Geneva: World Health Organization; 2012.
5. Briones JR, Talungchit P, Thavorncharoensap M, Chaikledkaew U. Economic evaluation of carbetocin as prophylaxis for postpartum hemorrhage in the Philippines. BMC Health Serv Res. 2020;20:975.
6. Lawrie TA, Rogozinska E, Sobiesuo P, Vogel JP, Ternent L, Oladapo OT. A systematic review of the cost-effectiveness of uterotonic agents for the prevention of postpartum hemorrhage. Int J Gynaecol Obstet. 2019;146(1):56-64.
7. Chao YS, McCormack S. Carbetocin for the Prevention of Post-Partum Hemorrhage: A Review of Clinical Effectiveness, Cost-Effectiveness, and Guidelines [Internet]. Ottawa (ON): Canadian Agency for Drugs and Technologies in Health; 2019.
8. Leduc D, Senikas V, Lalonde AB. No. 235-Active Management of the Third Stage of Labour: Prevention and Treatment of Postpartum Hemorrhage. J Obstet Gynaecol Can. 2018;40(12):e841-e855.
9. Mavrides E, Allard S, Chandraharan E, Collins P, Green L, Hunt BJ, et al.; on behalf of the Royal College of Obstetricians and Gynaecologists. Prevention and Management of Postpartum Haemorrhage: Green-top Guideline No. 52. BJOG. 2017;124(5):e106-e149.
10. Jin XH, Li D, Li X. Carbetocin vs oxytocin for prevention of postpartum hemorrhage after vaginal delivery: a meta-analysis. Medicine (Baltimore). 2019;98(47):e17911.
11. Albazee E, Alrashidi H, Laqwer R, Elmokid SR, Alghamdi WA, Almahmood H, et al. Intravenous Carbetocin Versus Rectal Misoprostol for the Active Management of the Third Stage of Labor: A Systematic Review and Meta-Analysis of Randomized Controlled Trials. Cureus. 2022;14(10):e30229.
12. Widmer M, Piaggio G, Nguyen TMH, Osoti A, Owa OO, Misra S, et al. WHO CHAMPION Trial Group. Heat-Stable Carbetocin versus Oxytocin to Prevent Hemorrhage after Vaginal Birth. N Engl J Med. 2018;379(8):743-52.
13. Tran NT, Bar-Zeev S, Zeck W, Schulte-Hillen C. Implementing Heat-Stable Carbetocin for Postpartum Haemorrhage Prevention in Low-Resource Settings: A Rapid Scoping Review. Int J Environ Res Public Health. 2022;19(7):3765.

CHAPTER 2

Ulipristal Acetate

Charmila Ayyavoo

■ BACKGROUND

Ulipristal acetate (UPA) is also known as CDB/VA-2914 and is a selective modulator of the progesterone receptor (PR). It is being increasingly used for the management of fibroids and as an emergency contraceptive. The drug needs to be used with caution because of severe side effects in some patients.

■ MODE OF ACTION

Ulipristal acetate is a selective progesterone receptor modulator (SPRM). SPRMs act on the PR. They can exhibit agonistic or antagonistic activity based on the tissue.

The main mode of action of ulipristal is on ovulation where it delays the rupture of the follicle. If given in the midfollicular phase, the drug can suppress the growth of the lead follicle. If administered in the luteal phase, it is known to decrease the thickness of the endometrium, delay the maturation, and alter the implantation markers, which are dependent on progesterone. This will cause reduced receptivity of the endometrium. All the above actions of ulipristal are useful for its usage as an emergency contraceptive.[1]

Progesterone is proposed to promote the growth of fibroids by two mechanisms. It causes upregulation of epidermal growth factor (EGF) and the *Bcl-2* gene. It also downregulates the tumor necrosis factor (TNF) gene. UPA is a progesterone antagonist and it blocks the proliferation of fibroid cells. It increases apoptotic activity by reducing the *Bcl-2* expression and increasing the cleaved caspase-3 expression in fibroid cells.[2]

Ulipristal acetate also suppresses neovascularization in fibroids by blocking vascular endothelial growth factor. This effect is seen only in fibroid cells and not in normal myometrial cells. It affects the tissue integrity of the fibroids by causing a reduction in collagen deposition in the extracellular spaces. This is due to the drug's action on metalloproteinases and collagen tissue.[3]

During therapy with UPA, there is no reduction in the basal levels of pituitary gonadotropins, and estradiol is present in the physiological range. Hence, symptoms of estrogen deficiency are not present during therapy with

UPA. The reason for amenorrhea during therapy is due to its action on the endometrial PRs. There is a relatively selective action of the drug, which is beneficial during therapy.[4] After stopping UPA, menstruation resumes in the patient within 4-5 weeks, but the reduction in size of the fibroids can be present for about 6 months.

USES

It is used in the management of fibroids based on its action as an antagonist in fibroid cells. It reduces menorrhagia in patients with fibroids. It is known to block progesterone pathways, which cause increase in the growth of fibroids and their maintenance. This leads to shrinking of fibroids.

The National Institute for Health and Care Excellence (NICE) guidelines advise UPA if surgery is unsafe or not necessary and when patient does not want to undergo surgery.[5] The PEARL trials show a reduction in abnormal uterine bleeding (AUB) and increase in quality of life with the usage of UPA. The trials also reveal a reduction in uterine size with UPA use.[6] The reduction in uterine and fibroid size is due to its antiproliferative, antifibrotic, and proapoptotic effects.

Ulipristal acetate can be used in the preoperative management of fibroids. A 3 months pretreatment increases the chances of complete resection. It also decreases the time of surgery and increases patient satisfaction 3 months after surgery.[7]

It is considered useful for women in the perimenopausal age group who want to avoid surgery. It is also useful in young women with fibroids who are symptomatic, but do not want to conceive. Surgery may be a problem if fibroids recur when they want to conceive. Medical therapy can be a temporizing method till they want to conceive. UPA is not useful for multiple, large fibroids. It does not cause the side effects of the commonly used gonadotropin-releasing hormone (GnRH) agonists such as hot flushes and loss of bone, which are due to the hypoestrogenic effect of the agonist preparation.

The other main use of the drug is for emergency contraception due to its effects on ovulation. If used within 120 hours of unprotected intercourse, UPA acts by inhibiting or delaying ovulation and stopping the endometrial proliferation.

It is being evaluated for providing continuous contraception by incorporating the drug in a vaginal ring. It is being tried for usage as an intrauterine contraceptive device such as the copper intrauterine system but with the incorporation of UPA instead of copper. The early results reveal that the device causes lesser menstrual bleeding compared to the copper device. The study also shows that there is a reduced incidence of PR modulation-associated changes in the endometrium and no incidence of adverse events. This use of UPA can be tried for patients who require long-acting contraception but are anemic.[8]

Ulipristal acetate has been compared with the levonorgestrel-releasing intrauterine system (LNG-IUS) in a trial for reducing heavy menstrual bleeding (HMB), irrespective of whether fibroids are present or not. The trial results reveal that both are of equal efficacy for reducing HMB. UPA induces amenorrhea more effectively than LNG-IUS.[9]

It is known to reduce cell viability and growth in Ishikawa endometrial cancer cells. A combination of UPA with an antagonist of estrogen receptors is seen to downregulate proinflammatory cytokines in endometrial cells, which showed cancerous change. There is ongoing research to determine whether UPA can influence inflammatory changes in endometrial cancer due to its effect on the endogenous secretion of estrogen.[10]

Ulipristal acetate can be used in preoperative treatment for adenomyosis. It can correct anemia before surgery but cannot be used as long-term treatment because of the side effects on the liver.[11]

■ SIDE EFFECTS

Side effects associated commonly with UPA are gastrointestinal symptoms such as nausea, vomiting, dryness of the oral cavity and throat, loose stools, disorders of appetite, flatulence, disturbed taste, and thirst. The user can also suffer from headaches, backache, body pain, pelvic pain, mastalgia, irregular menstruation, altered mood, and dizziness. Side effects such as fever, chills, hot flashes, drowsiness, impaired concentration, disorders of vision, insomnia, dermatitis, and vulval disorders are unusual. Redness of the eyes, gritty sensation in the eyes, fainting attacks, tremors, vertigo, perineal itching, dyspareunia, and rupture of ovarian cysts are rare complications of the drug.[12]

The dangerous side effect of UPA is the causation of acute hepatitis. It can rarely cause acute liver failure with the need for a liver transplantation. 765,000 patients were treated with UPA. Eight patients had severe liver injury.[13] In 2018, the European Medicines Agency (EMA) advised liver function screening for all users of UPA for fibroids. This was advised pretreatment, during treatment, and after treatment. In March 2020, UPA use was suspended by EMA as five more cases of hepatic damage were reported. On 12th November 2020, the EMA has advised to restrict the use of the drug. It has recommended the drug for premenopausal women for whom surgical procedures are contraindicated or other methods are not working.[14]

Liver function tests are done after 2 months of therapy and repeated whenever deemed necessary.[5]

Ulipristal acetate can cause thickening of the endometrial layer due to the endogenous estrogen release. This is called progesterone receptor modulator-associated endometrial changes (PAEC). This is a benign pathology, which is reversible on stopping the drug. They differ from the changes in hyperplasia of the endometrium and cancer of the endometrium. In histology, the changes identified due to the drug are cystic dilatation of the glands, distortion of the epithelium, apoptosis, and mitotic activity, which is low grade in the glands and stroma. The mechanisms by which these changes happen and their significance have not been fully understood.[15]

■ DOSAGES ADVISED

Ulipristal acetate is advised at a dosage of 5–10 mg/day for the management of menorrhagia due to fibroids. UPA 10 mg dose is more beneficial in inducing amenorrhea, but safety profile is better with the 5 mg dose.[16]

It can be used preoperatively in fibroids management or can be used intermittently as 3-month courses. 3-month courses are advisable as PAEC in the endometrium can reverse after the stoppage of therapy. According to NICE guidelines, UPA needs to be given as a 5-g dose daily for 3 months up to four courses of therapy. It can be given if the fibroid is <3 cm in diameter and the patient is anemic.[5]

At a single dose of 30 mg, UPA is used as an emergency contraceptive. It needs to be used within 120 hours of unprotected intercourse.

■ CONCLUSION

Ulipristal acetate is a drug that can be useful in women with symptomatic fibroids and as an emergency contraceptive. When it is used continuously in the treatment of fibroids, it can cause severe complications such as hepatitis in a small group of patients. If adequate monitoring is done during therapy and the drug is administered in intermittent doses, UPA has a place in the management of fibroids. It will be especially useful when a short course of therapy is needed for symptomatic relief.

■ REFERENCES

1. Jadav SP, Parmar DM. Ulipristal acetate, a progesterone receptor modulator for emergency contraception. J Pharmacol Pharmacother. 2012;3(2):109-11.
2. Maruo T, Matsuo H, Samoto T, Shimomura Y, Kurachi O, Gao Z. Effects of progesterone on uterine leiomyoma growth and apoptosis. Steroids. 2000;65(10-11):585-92.
3. Courtoy GE, Henriet P, Marbaix E, de Codt M, Luyckx M, Donnez J. Matrix metalloproteinase activity correlates with uterine myoma volume reduction after ulipristal acetate treatment. J Clin Endocrinol Metab. 2018;103(4):1566-73.
4. Spitz IM. Clinical utility of progesterone receptor modulators and their effect on the endometrium. Curr Opin Obstet Gynecol. 2009;21(4):318-24.
5. National Institute for Health Care and Excellence. (2018). Heavy menstrual bleeding: assessment and management. [online] Available from https://www.

nice.org.uk/guidance/ng88/resources/heavy-menstrual-bleeding-assessment-and-management-pdf-1837701412549. [Last accessed August, 2023].
6. Donnez J, Vázquez F, Tomaszewski J, Nouri K, Bouchard P, Fauser BC. Long-term treatment of uterine fibroids with ulipristal acetate. Fertil Steril. 2014;101(6):1565-73.
7. Ferrero S, Racca A, Tafi E, Alessandri F, Venturini PL, Leone Roberti Maggiore U. Ulipristal Acetate Before High Complexity Hysteroscopic Myomectomy: A Retrospective Comparative Study. J Minim Invasive Gynecol. 2016;23(3):390-5.
8. Brache V, Vieira CS, Plagianos M, Lansiaux M, Merkatz R, Sussman H. Pharmacodynamics and pharmacokinetics of a copper intrauterine contraceptive system releasing ulipristal acetate: a randomized proof-of-concept study. Contraception. 2021;104(4):327-36.
9. Whitaker LHR, Middleton LJ, Daniels JP, Williams ARW, Priest L, Odedra S. Ulipristal acetate versus levonorgestrel-releasing intrauterine system for heavy menstrual bleeding (UCON): a randomised controlled phase III trial. EClinicalMedicine. 2023;60:101995.
10. Kanda R, Miyagawa Y, Wada-Hiraike O, Hiraike H, Nagasaka K, Ryo E. Ulipristal acetate simultaneously provokes antiproliferative and proinflammatory responses in endometrial cancer cells. Heliyon. 2021;8(1):e08696.
11. Capmas P, Brun JL, Legendre G, Koskas M, Merviel P, Fernandez H. Ulipristal acetate use in adenomyosis: a randomized controlled trial. J Gynecol Obstet Hum Reprod. 2021;50(1):101978.
12. Donnez J, Courtoy GE, Donnez O, Dolmans MM. Ulipristal acetate for the management of large uterine fibroids associated with heavy bleeding: a review. Reprod Biomed Online. 2018;37(2):216-23.
13. Meunier L, Meszaros M, Pageaux GP, Delay JM, Herrero A, Pinzani V. Acute liver failure requiring transplantation caused by ulipristal acetate. Clin Res in Hepatology Gastroenterol. 2020;44(3):e45-9.
14. European Medicines Agency. Esmya Article-20 procedure—Scientific conclusions. [online] Available from https://www.ema.europa.eu/en/documents/referral/esmya-article-20-procedure-scientific-conclusions_en.pdf. [Last accessed August, 2023].
15. De Milliano I, Van Hattum D, Ket JCF, Huirne JAF, Hehenkamp WJK. Endometrial changes during ulipristal acetate use: a systematic review. Eur J Obstet Gynecol Reprod Bio. 2017;214:56-64.
16. Kounidas G, Kastora SL, Barnott E, Black L, Robinson-Burke T, Gould A. Efficacy of ulipristal acetate in women with fibroid induced menorrhagia: a systematic review and meta-analysis. J Gynecol Obstet Hum Reprod. 2021;50(9):102173.

CHAPTER 3

Dydrogesterone

Bhaskar Pal, Poushali Sanyal, Sujoy Dasgupta

■ BACKGROUND

Progesterone is a steroid hormone produced by the corpus luteum, which is responsible for the maintenance of pregnancy. It is a progesterone and is approved for clinical use in a variety of conditions associated with progesterone deficiency. Dydrogesterone is synthesized in the laboratory by stereoisomerization of progesterone. Structurally, dydrogesterone (6-dehydro-retroprogesterone) is a retroprogesterone, where the orientation of side chains of carbon 9 and carbon 10 is altered (carbon 9 is having hydrogen in the β-orientation and carbon 10 contains methyl group in the α-orientation). There is an additional double bond at carbon 6, creating a "bent" structure, responsible for higher affinity for progesterone receptors.[1]

■ PHARMACOLOGY

Owing to its limited bioavailability through the oral route, extensive hepatic first-pass metabolism and the risk of intrahepatic cholestasis, micronized progesterone should preferably be administered by vaginal, intramuscular, or subcutaneous routes. In contrast, because of the structural changes, the oral bioavailability of dydrogesterone is better than that of micronized progesterone. Additionally, dydrogesterone does not interact with glucocorticoid, mineralocorticoid, androgen, or estrogen receptors, thereby minimizing the adverse effects on the fetus.[2]

As a result, secretory transformation of the endometrium occurs with dydrogesterone at a dose 10–20 times lower than that with micronized progesterone (10 mg vs. 200 mg). The requirement of low dose can account for the minimal side effects of dydrogesterone and less risk of altered liver function.[3]

■ IMMUNOMODULATION

In addition to providing support to pregnancy by the decidualization of the endometrium and maintaining uterine quiescence, progesterones also exert immunomodulatory action by synthesis of progesterone-induced blocking factor (PIBF). This in turn shifts immune system to T helper cell 2 response (Th2) from T helper cell 1 response (Th1), resulting in tolerance of the fetus which is regarded as "semi-allogeneic tissue". Dydrogesterone exerts better immunomodulatory actions than natural progesterone. In addition, dydrogesterone, like other progestogens, lowers subendometrial vascular resistance by promoting nitric oxide synthesis and thereby plays important role in supplying oxygen and nutrients to the embryos. This is also a crucial step in maintenance of pregnancy.[4,5]

LUTEAL PHASE SUPPORT IN ASSISTED REPRODUCTIVE TECHNOLOGY

In assisted reproductive technology (ART) cycles, luteal phase support is essential because of several reasons:
- Pituitary downregulation by gonadotropin-releasing hormone (GnRH) agonists and antagonists can suppress luteinizing hormone (LH) secretion essential for maintenance of corpus luteum.
- Disruption of granulose cells during ovum pick-up can remove a portion of the source of progesterone.
- Human chorionic gonadotropin (hCG) used for trigger can cause short-loop feedback inhibition on pituitary LH.
- Supraphysiological levels of gonadal steroids secreted from the hyperstimulated ovaries can suppress pituitary LH.

In addition, in frozen embryo transfer (FET) cycles, where exogenous estrogen is given for endometrial priming, there is no functional corpus luteum. Hence, luteal phase support is necessary. Options include progesterone, hCG, and GnRH agonists. A Cochrane review found that while hCG and progesterone have the same efficacy, use of hCG is associated with increased risk of ovarian hyperstimulation syndrome (OHSS). Addition of GnRH agonists to progesterone seems to improve the outcome, but stronger evidence is required to support this in routine practice. Therefore, progesterone is the "standard" and mainstay of luteal phase support.[6,7]

Regarding progesterone used for luteal phase support, different forms are available. Intramuscular progesterone provides reliable and adequate plasma concentration of the drug but is limited by pain, abscess formation and therefore, poor compliance. The subcutaneous route is an alternative but is limited by lack of adequate number of studies. Vaginal progesterone in the form of tablet, pessary, and gel is associated with good bioavailability, because it has a "first uterine pass" phenomenon, by which it delivers high concentration of drug to the uterus. However, it is associated with discomfort and vaginal discharge.

Progesterone should be started on the day of oocyte retrieval in fresh transfer cycle and in case of FET cycle when the endometrial thickness is

>7 mm. As per convention, progesterone should be continued till end of first trimester, when luteoplacental shift occurs and placenta becomes autonomous in secreting progesterone. However, there is some evidence that progesterone can be stopped after a positive pregnancy test result, because the growing blastocyst secretes hCG, which can provide support to the corpus luteum to secrete endogenous progesterone in early pregnancy.[8]

The first randomized trial between oral dydrogesterone and vaginal progesterone conducted in India in 2002–2003 found that both of these drugs had similar efficacy in terms of successful pregnancies, but patient satisfaction was better with oral dydrogesterone. In addition, there was no difference in alteration of liver function between these two groups.[9]

The LOTUS I trial was a multicentric randomized placebo-controlled trial between oral dydrogesterone and vaginal micronized progesterone on 1,031 subjects, which showed that pregnancy rates and live birth rates were similar between two groups. Similarly, the LOTUS II trial was a randomized trial between oral dydrogesterone and intravaginal progesterone gel, which also yielded similar results. All these trials included women undergoing fresh transfers only. Interestingly, one meta-analysis found that dydrogesterone was associated with even better pregnancy rate and live birth rate compared to vaginal progesterone in fresh transfer cycles.[10-12]

Regarding FET cycles, one randomized study found that oral dydrogesterone and vaginal progesterone had similar efficacy but the former was better tolerated. Finally, a meta-analysis that included both fresh and frozen transfer cycles found that oral dydrogesterone had "at least similar" like vaginal progesterone. The guideline formulated by the European Society of Human Reproduction and Embryology (ESHRE) suggested dydrogesterone as one of the options for luteal phase support. There is some evidence that dydrogesterone is also effective for luteal phase support in intrauterine insemination (IUI) cycles.[13-15]

SUPPRESSION OF LUTEINIZING HORMONE IN ASSISTED REPRODUCTIVE TECHNOLOGY

In ART cycles, suppression of premature LH surge is important to prevent premature ovulation and to prevent the harmful effects of elevated LH on oocytes. Conventionally, GnRH agonists and antagonists are used for this purpose. The role of progesterone for prevention of the LH surge has been investigated as an alternative to GnRH analogs. Dydrogesterone possibly does not inhibit ovulation in the usual therapeutic doses. However, at a dose of 20 mg it can suppress LH surge. Some evidence support the theory that dydrogesterone could be as efficacious as GnRH antagonists in suppressing LH in IVF cycles. Oral dydrogesterone was similarly effective like natural micronized progesterone or medroxyprogesterone acetate in the prevention of premature LH surge in IVF cycles. Such usage can reduce the overall cost of the treatment.[16,17]

■ THREATENED MISCARRIAGE

Threatened miscarriage occurs in 20% of all pregnancies worldwide and is diagnosed when vaginal bleeding occurs with or without abdominal pain during the first 5 months of pregnancy. It is clinically diagnosed by the following prerequisites—a closed cervical os and a viable intrauterine fetus. Unfortunately, without any intervention, almost half of threatened miscarriages ultimately end in an inevitable miscarriage. Progesterone induces uterine quiescence and is commonly used to treat threatened abortions. Initially oral, intramuscular, and natural micronized vaginal progesterone were commonly used to treat threatened miscarriage. Their side effects observed were drowsiness, nausea, and vomiting. This led to the emergence of dydrogesterone to treat threatened miscarriage.

Studies have shown that vaginally administered natural micronized progesterone and oral dydrogesterone are equally effective in the treatment of threatened miscarriage. In the Indian context, patients prefer oral dydrogesterone to vaginal progesterone as in a tropical country, vaginal application of progesterone becomes cumbersome and reduces patient compliance. The dosage of oral dydrogesterone as per ESHRE guidelines is 40 mg orally as a stat dose followed by 30 mg orally per day (divided as 10 mg orally thrice daily) until the bleeding stops. A maintenance dose of 10 mg twice daily till 20 weeks of pregnancy is recommended.[18,19]

There are various mechanisms by which dydrogesterone effectively prevents miscarriage. It reduces the release of various proinflammatory cytokines from the uterine myometrium and placenta. It also shifts the cytokine cascade toward the Th2 helper cells through the enhanced release of PIBF, which promotes uterine quiescence. Many recent studies have reported several beneficial effects of dydrogesterone in threatened miscarriage. In one study, 146 women presenting with varying degrees of vaginal bleeding during the first 3 months of pregnancy were randomized to two groups. One group received 10 mg oral dydrogesterone twice daily ($n = 86$), while the other group received no treatment ($n = 60$). The incidence of miscarriage was observed to be 17.5% in the group receiving dydrogesterone, whereas in the other group it was 25% ($p < 0.05$).[20]

■ RECURRENT MISCARRIAGE

Recurrent miscarriage is defined as two or more consecutive spontaneous pregnancy losses within 20 weeks of pregnancy. Recurrent miscarriage is both physically and emotionally challenging for the couples, and in 50% of the cases, no causative factor can be identified. The incidence of recurrent miscarriage is 1.5-2%. It is often seen that immunological factors play a key role in causing recurrent spontaneous pregnancy losses, followed by other factors such as genetic factors or antiphospholipid antibody syndrome. Women with recurrent miscarriages are often found to have lower serum progesterone levels. Dydrogesterone has better bioavailability and patient tolerance with minimal side effects. Hence, it is recommended by ESHRE for the prevention of recurrent miscarriages.[21]

Immunomodulation via the reduction of Th1 cells, upregulation of Th2 cells, and production of PIBF in the trophoblast helps in successful continuation of pregnancy. Studies have shown that women being treated with dydrogesterone had increased levels of serum progesterone and hCG and had a higher chance of a successful pregnancy. The ESHRE recommended dosage of dydrogesterone in treatment of recurrent miscarriage is 10 mg twice daily orally from onset of pregnancy till 20 completed weeks of pregnancy. Studies have showed similar live birth rates in women treated for recurrent miscarriage with dydrogesterone and vaginal micronized progesterone. Thus, dydrogesterone orally is a safe and efficacious treatment for recurrent miscarriage.[22,23]

■ EMERGING APPLICATIONS

Dydrogesterone has emerged as a useful agent in the treatment of secondary amenorrhea, dysfunctional uterine bleeding, endometriosis, endometrial carcinoma, and prevention of preterm birth. However, further studies are required before clinically establishing its role in these areas.[24]

■ SAFETY CONCERNS

Based on a "semi-systematic review" of 32 clinical studies, dydrogesterone was found to be well tolerated during its use over the last six decades for various indications. In the context of ART, vaginal bleeding, irritation, and sexual difficulties were less encountered with dydrogesterone compared to vaginal progesterone. However, some minor side effects such as nausea, flatulence, headache, and abdominal pain appeared to be more common. In the context of menopausal hormone therapy, the risk of breast and endometrial cancer, venous thromboembolism, and cardiovascular events were found to be minimal.[25]

Regarding use in early pregnancy, a case-control study on more than 400 infants born in the Gaza strip was published in 2015. It found positive correlation between dydrogesterone exposure in early pregnancy and congenital cardiac diseases in the offspring [odds ratio (OR) 2.71; 95% confidence interval (CI) 1.54-4.24]. However, this study was criticized owing to lack of adherence to the basic principles of epidemiological research. It did not match for confounding factors like previous miscarriage (which itself increases the risk of congenital cardiac disease) and relied on recall data, rather than medical records. Hence, no clear causal relationship could be established from this study.[26]

An individual participant data meta-analysis did not find any increased incidence of adverse obstetric outcome or congenital anomalies in pregnancies exposed to dydrogesterone. Similarly, other authors concluded the same in review and meta-analysis. In fact the LOTUS I and LOTUS II trials could not find any increased incidence of congenital anomalies in babies exposed to dydrogesterone in utero. Therefore, dydrogesterone can safely be used before and during pregnancy.[27]

■ CONCLUSION

Dydrogesterone is an essential tool in the armamentarium of obstetricians, gynecologists, and reproductive endocrinologists. It has a wide variety of evidence-based applications, while more use case scenarios are being explored even today. It is proven to be beneficial in ART, threatened and recurrent miscarriage, and recently in endometriosis. It is safe, effective, and is widely available in India having been relaunched in a cost-effective fashion.

■ REFERENCES

1. Griesinger G, Tournaye H, Macklon N, Petraglia F, Arck P, Blockeel C, et al. Dydrogesterone: pharmacological profile and mechanism of action as luteal phase support in assisted reproduction. Reprod Biomed Online. 2019;38(2):249-59.
2. Stanczyk FZ, Hapgood JP, Winer S, Mishell DR Jr. Progestogens used in postmenopausal hormone therapy: differences in their pharmacological properties, intracellular actions, and clinical effects. Endocr Rev. 2013; 34(2):171-208.
3. Ghabril M, Chalasani N, Björnsson E. Drug-induced liver injury: a clinical update. Curr Opin Gastroenterol. 2010;26(3):222-6.
4. Szekeres-Bartho J, Barakonyi A, Par G, Polgar B, Palkovics T, Szereday L. Progesterone as an immunomodulatory molecule. Int Immunopharmacol. 2001;1(6):1037-48.
5. Ghosh S, Chattopadhyay R, Goswami S, Chaudhury K, Chakravarty B, Ganesh A. Assessment of sub-endometrial blood flow parameters following dydrogesterone and micronized vaginal progesterone administration in women with idiopathic recurrent miscarriage: a pilot study. J Obstet Gynaecol Res. 2014;40(7):1871-6.
6. van der Linden M, Buckingham K, Farquhar C, Kremer JA, Metwally M. Luteal phase support for assisted reproduction cycles. Cochrane Database Syst Rev. 2011;(10):CD009154.
7. Gayet V, Vasilopulos I, de Ziengler D. Luteal-phase support in assisted reproductive technology. In: Gardner DK, Weissman A, Howles CM, Shoham Z. (Eds). Textbook of Assisted Reproductive Techniques, 5th edition. Florida: Taylor & Francis Group. 2018. pp. 612-7.

8. Watters M, Noble M, Child T, Nelson S. Short versus extended progesterone supplementation for luteal phase support in fresh IVF cycles: a systematic review and meta-analysis. Reprod Biomed Online. 2020;40(1):143-50.
9. Chakravarty BN, Shirazee HH, Dam P, Goswami SK, Chatterjee R, Ghosh S. Oral dydrogesterone versus intravaginal micronised progesterone as luteal phase support in assisted reproductive technology (ART) cycles: results of a randomised study. J Steroid Biochem Mol Biol. 2005;97(5):416-20.
10. Tournaye H, Sukhikh GT, Kahler E, Griesinger G. A Phase III randomized controlled trial comparing the efficacy, safety and tolerability of oral dydrogesterone versus micronized vaginal progesterone for luteal support in in vitro fertilization. Hum Reprod. 2017;32(5):1019-27.
11. Griesinger G, Blockeel C, Sukhikh GT, Patki A, Dhorepatil B, Yang DZ, et al. Oral dydrogesterone versus intravaginal micronized progesterone gel for luteal phase support in IVF: a randomized clinical trial. Hum Reprod. 2018;33(12):2212-21.
12. Griesinger G, Blockeel C, Kahler E, Pexman-Fieth C, Olofsson JI, Driessen S, et al. Dydrogesterone as an oral alternative to vaginal progesterone for IVF luteal phase support: a systematic review and individual participant data meta-analysis. PLoS One. 2020;15(11):e0241044.
13. Barbosa MWP, Valadares NPB, Barbosa ACP, Amaral AS, Iglesias JR, Nastri CO, et al. Oral dydrogesterone vs. vaginal progesterone capsules for luteal-phase support in women undergoing embryo transfer: a systematic review and meta-analysis. JBRA Assist Reprod. 2018;22(2):148-56.
14. Bosch E, Broer S, Griesinger G, Grynberg M, Humaidan P, Kolibianakis E, et al.; Ovarian Stimulation TEGGO. ESHRE guideline: ovarian stimulation for IVF/ICSI. Hum Reprod Open. 2020;2020(2):hoaa009.
15. Gün İ, Özdamar Ö, Yılmaz A. Luteal phase support in intrauterine insemination cycles. Turk J Obstet Gynecol. 2016;13(2):90-4.
16. Gurbuz AS, Gode F. Dydrogesterone-primed ovarian stimulation is an effective alternative to gonadotropin-releasing hormone antagonist protocol for freeze-all cycles in polycystic ovary syndrome. J Obstet Gynaecol Res. 2020;46(8):1403-11.
17. Yu S, Long H, Chang HY, Liu Y, Gao H, Zhu J, et al. New application of dydrogesterone as a part of a progestin-primed ovarian stimulation protocol for IVF: a randomized controlled trial including 516 first IVF/ICSI cycles. Hum Reprod. 2018;33(2):229-37.
18. Mirza FG, Patki A, Pexman-Fieth C. Dydrogesterone use in early pregnancy. Gynecol Endocrinol. 2016;32:97-106.
19. Schindler AE. Progestational effects of dydrogesterone in vitro, in vivo and on the human endometrium. Maturitas. 2009;65:S3-11.
20. Wong LF, Porter TF, Scott JR. Immunotherapy for recurrent miscarriage. Cochrane Database Syst Rev. 2014;CD000112.
21. Li XN, Zhang PY, Hui XL. Comparison of the effect of dydrogesterone and progesterone in unexplained recurrent miscarriage. Guizhou Medical Journal. 2020;44:1739-40.
22. Raghupathy R, Al Mutawa E, Makhseed M, Azizieh F, Szekeres-Bartho J. Modulation of cytokine production by dydrogesterone in lymphocytes from women with recurrent miscarriage. BJOG. 2005;112:1096-101.
23. Kumar A, Begum N, Prasad S, Aggarwal S, Sharma S. Oral dydrogesterone treatment during early pregnancy to prevent recurrent pregnancy loss and

its role in modulation of cytokine production: a double-blind, randomized, parallel, placebo-controlled trial. Fertil Steril. 2014;102:1357-1363.e3.
24. EPPPIC Group. Evaluating Progestogens for Preventing Preterm birth International Collaborative (EPPPIC): meta-analysis of individual participant data from randomised controlled trials. Lancet. 2021;397:1183-94.
25. Ott J, Egarter C, Aguilera A. Dydrogesterone after 60 years: a glance at the safety profile. Gynecol Endocrinol. 2022;38(4):279-87.
26. Zaqout M, Aslem E, Abuqamar M, Abughazza O, Panzer J, De Wolf D, et al. The impact of oral intake of dydrogesterone on fetal heart development during early pregnancy. Pediatr Cardiol. 2015;36(7):1483-8.
27. Katalinic A, Shulman LP, Strauss JF, Garcia-Velasco JA, van den Anker JN. A critical appraisal of safety data on dydrogesterone for the support of early pregnancy: a scoping review and meta-analysis. Reprod Biomed Online. 2022;45(2):365-73.

CHAPTER 4

Dehydroepiandrosterone (DHEA)

Nandita Palshetkar, Pratik Tambe

■ BACKGROUND

Dehydroepiandrosterone (DHEA) is a naturally occurring hormone produced in the human adrenal glands, specifically in the reticular zone of the suprarenal cortex and also in the ovarian theca cells. It is a precursor to both testosterone and estrogen and plays a significant role in normal reproductive health. Over the past decade, DHEA supplementation has gained momentum in the field of fertility treatment. It has been extensively studied in assisted reproduction in women with poor ovarian reserve (POR). This chapter aims to explore the potential benefits, mechanisms of action, and controversies surrounding the use of DHEA in in vitro fertilization (IVF).

■ IN VITRO FERTILIZATION

In vitro fertilization is a widely used assisted reproductive technology that involves the collection of mature eggs from a woman's ovaries, which are then fertilized with sperm in a laboratory setting outside the body. The resulting embryos, which grow over the next 2–3 or 5 days, are transferred back into the woman's uterus. While IVF has revolutionized fertility treatment by aiding conception for many couples, the success rates are still variable. Various

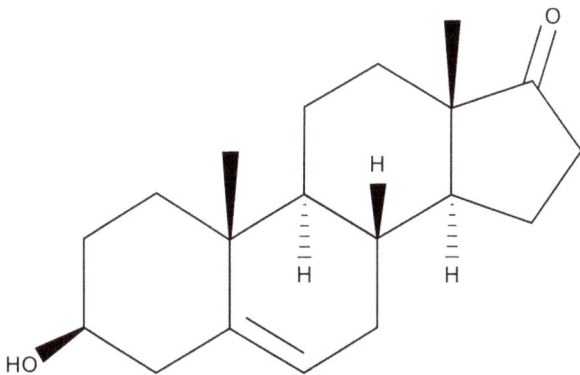

Fig. 1: Dehydroepiandrosterone (DHEA) structure.

factors affect the success of IVF, including the age of the woman, underlying the complexity of the fertility issues and the quality of the embryos. Retrieval of fewer oocytes is associated with a lower number of embryos for transfer and a lower success rate. POR frequency is estimated at 5-18% for IVF/intracytoplasmic sperm injection (ICSI) cycles, with a pregnancy rate as low as 2-4%.[1,2]

ROLE OF DEHYDROEPIANDROSTERONE IN FERTILITY

Dehydroepiandrosterone is essential for optimal ovarian function, and its levels decline naturally with age. Research suggests that DHEA supplementation may help improve fertility outcomes by enhancing ovarian response and increasing both the quality and quantity of eggs retrieved during IVF treatment. DHEA is an androgen precursor, which supports the growth and maturation of ovarian follicles and potentially aids in the production of healthier oocytes.

MECHANISMS OF ACTION

The precise mechanisms through which DHEA exerts its beneficial effects in IVF are not fully understood. However, several theories exist. DHEA may act by improving the ovarian microenvironment and increasing the sensitivity of the ovaries to exogenous gonadotropin stimulation, enhancing follicular development and promoting healthier egg and embryo quality. Oral administration of DHEA increases serum levels of insulin-like growth factor 1 (IGF-1), which has a positive effect on follicular development and oocyte quality. Hence, precycle DHEA supplementation has been extensively studied in women with diminished ovarian reserve (DOR) or POR to treatment.

ALTERED GENE EXPRESSION

One of the important steps for oocyte maturation depends on the connection between oocytes and cumulus cells (CCs). Hence, changes in the gene expression of CCs in women with POR following DHEA supplementation could potentially promote oocyte maturation. It has been demonstrated that the expression levels of *PTGS2*, *HAS2*, and *GREM1* genes are associated with morphological and physiological features. In addition, the gene expression profile of metabolic (*PFKP*), signaling (*PTGS2* and *GREM1*), and extracellular matrix (ECM; *VCAN*) components in CC masses could serve as indicators for oocytes with elevated developmental potential, which may result in improved implantation rates.[3]

The expression level of *VCAN* in CCs exhibits a positive correlation with early embryo morphology scores. This could also be utilized to evaluate oocyte developmental competence, supplementing traditional embryological morphological assessments. Nine genes in CCs of recruited women have been shown to be significantly different after DHEA supplementation. Three of the genes (*HAS2*, *VCAN*, and *THBS1*)—involved in ECM formation—are upregulated. Inversely, three genes (*RUNX2*, *CBX 3*, and *TRIM 28*) related to cell development and differentiation upregulation are downregulated.[4]

■ CELLULAR APOPTOSIS

Apoptosis, a biologically significant and genetically regulated form of cell death, plays a crucial role in ovarian function and oocyte development. Upon the transmission of stress stimuli to the mitochondria, proapoptotic members of the *BCL-2* family, *BAX* and *BAK*, enhance the mitochondrial membrane's permeability to proteins like cytochrome c. Two genes related to apoptosis regulation, namely *BCL-2* and *BAX*, have shown lower expression levels, but their ratio significantly increased.

■ MITOCHONDRIAL FUNCTION

In women with a POR, DHEA supplementation leads to a decrease in the mRNA levels of *BAX, BAD,* caspase-3, caspase-9, and cytochrome c in CCs. This correlates with a reduced percentage of apoptotic cells when compared to the nonsupplemented POR women.

TFAM is an important protein that binds to mitochondrial DNA (mtDNA) and modulates mitochondrial transcription initiation, serving as a key regulator of mtDNA copy number. *TFAM* gene expression, mitochondrial dehydrogenase activity, and mitochondrial mass were found to be elevated in CCs after DHEA supplementation. This result suggests that DHEA supplementation positively affects the mitochondrial function of CCs.[5,6]

■ SENESCENCE AND AGING

Cellular senescence is characterized by the irreversible suppression of cell proliferation in response to various stressors. The SA-β-gal activity, characterized as β-gal activity detectable at pH 6.0 in senescent cells, is used as a senescence biomarker due to the simplicity of the assay technique and its apparent specificity for senescent cells. The senescent phenotype of CCs exhibited improvement in older patients following DHEA supplementations. There was a significantly lower percentage of SA-β-gal-positive CCs in comparison to the group that did not receive DHEA supplementation. DHEA could therefore be a therapeutic agent utilized for delaying ovarian aging and enhancing oocyte yield and quality.[7]

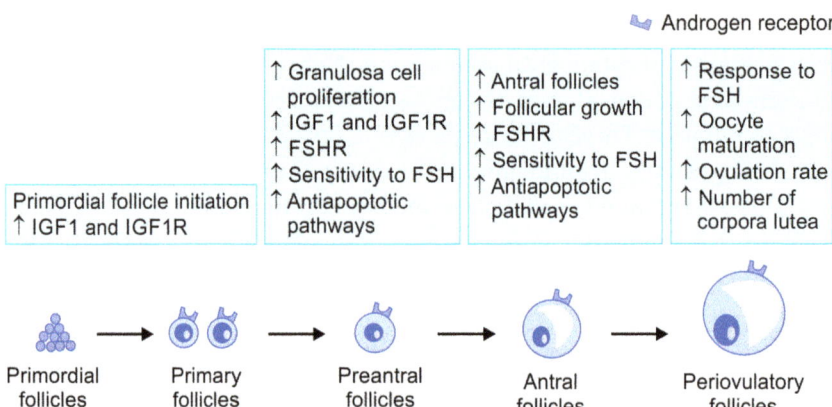

Fig. 2: Androgen effects on folliculogenesis.[8] (FSH: follicle-stimulating hormone; FSHR: follicle-stimulating hormone receptor; GF1: growth factor 1; IGF1R: insulin-like growth factor 1 receptor)

■ DOSAGE AND TREATMENT DURATION

The optimal dosage and treatment duration of DHEA supplementation remain topics of debate. A daily dose of 25–75 mg is recommended with a treatment duration of at least 3 months before undergoing IVF treatment. Individualized approaches are crucial, and it is essential to consult with a medical professional experienced in fertility treatment for personalized dosing and monitoring.

■ CLINICAL EVIDENCE

Numerous studies have investigated the effects of DHEA supplementation on IVF outcomes, although findings thus far have been inconclusive. Some studies have reported positive effects, such as increased pregnancy rates and improved embryo quality, while others have found no significant impact. Different definitions, inclusion criteria, variations in study protocols, patient demographics, and DHEA dosage, timing, and duration of therapy may contribute to the disagreements observed in research. In future, well-designed randomized controlled trials (RCTs) are necessary to generate more definitive conclusions.

Out of 68 studies, 5 RCTs fulfilled the inclusion criteria in a meta-analysis performed in 2018. They included studies that considered POR by the presence of at least two of the three following Bologna criteria: (1) patients older than 40 years of age; (2) antral follicle count lower than 5, or decreased antimüllerian hormone (AMH); and (c) a deficient prior ovarian response.[1-9]

The meta-analysis had data from 910 patients who underwent IVF/ICSI, of which 413 had received DHEA. DHEA use was associated with a significant increase in pregnancy likelihood [odds ratio (OR) 1.8, 95% CI (confidence interval) 1.29-2.51, and $p = 0.001$]. The use of DHEA was associated with a significant reduction in the likelihood of abortion (OR 0.25, 95% CI 0.07-0.95, and $p = 0.045$). There was no association between DHEA use and the number of oocytes retrieved [standardized mean difference (SMD) −0.01, 95% CI −0.16-0.13, and $p < 0.05$].[1]

■ LARGEST META-ANALYSIS AND SYSTEMATIC REVIEW

A Human Reproduction Update published in 2020 identified 1,124 studies, of which 46 trials reporting on 6,312 women were included in the systematic review. Another 19 trials defining POR using the Bologna criteria with 2,677 women were included in the network meta-analysis. Compared with controls, DHEA treatments resulted in a significantly higher chance of clinical pregnancy (OR 2.46, 95% CI 1.16-5.23). Considering the number of embryos transferred, testosterone treatment led to the highest number of embryos transferred [weighted mean difference (WMD) 0.72, 0.11-1.33].

Dehydroepiandrosterone, coenzyme Q10 (CoQ10), and growth hormone (GH) were the top three agents that improved the probability of achieving pregnancy, and these treatments also required lower dosages of gonadotropins compared to controls and had lower cycle cancellation rates in patients with POR. They concluded that supplementation with adjuvant treatment during controlled ovarian stimulation (COS) is the optimal management for patients with POR.[10]

■ CONTROVERSIES TO CONSENSUS

Despite some promising results, the use of DHEA in IVF is not without controversy. Critics argue that more research is required before widespread adoption, highlighting concerns regarding potential side effects and the unknown long-term effects of DHEA supplementation. Additionally, DHEA is classified as a controlled substance in some countries, limiting its accessibility.

The current European Society of Human Reproduction and Embryology (ESHRE) guideline on ovarian stimulation (OS) for IVF/ICSI published in 2020 does not recommend adjuvant therapy with DHEA. Use of DHEA before and/or during OS is probably not recommended for poor responders (conditional 3/4).[11]

The T-TRANSPORT (Testosterone TRANSdermal Gel for Poor Ovarian Responders Trial), which is currently underway, has an intervention group receiving 5.5 mg daily transdermal testosterone for 2 months prior to an IVF cycle and powered with clinical pregnancy rate as the primary outcome measure. This trial is expected to complete by 2024 and will help clarify the role of androgens in IVF.[12]

■ DIRECTIONS FOR FUTURE RESEARCH[5]

Future studies should consider incorporating the following elements in their study design to generate more robust evidence:
- Stratification, to reduce potential bias and increase the statistical power of the study
- Personalized treatment approaches, including identifying key genetic markers that predict response and tailoring treatment accordingly
- Multicenter collaboration, which can help increase the study population
- Integration of -omics technologies, where it could lead to a better understanding of the underlying molecular mechanisms and help in the development of more targeted and effective interventions.

■ CONCLUSION

Dehydroepiandrosterone holds promise as an adjunct therapy for women undergoing IVF treatment, particularly those with DOR and poor response to stimulation. While research regarding DHEA supplementation and IVF outcomes continues to evolve, different trials report varying outcomes. Therefore, it is crucial for patients considering DHEA supplementation to consult with experienced fertility clinicians for individualized advice and to carefully weigh the potential benefits and risks associated with its use.

The largest meta-analysis so far has identified that DHEA supplementation results in a significantly better number of high-quality embryos being transferred, leading to a higher chance of clinical pregnancy. DHEA-pretreated women also required lower dosages of gonadotropins compared to controls and had lower cycle cancellation rates. More well-designed clinical trials are necessary to establish the role of androgens, including DHEA in IVF, and determine their place in fertility treatment protocols.

■ REFERENCES

1. Schwarze JE, Canales J, Crosby J, Ortega-Hrepich C, Villa S, Pommer R. DHEA use to improve likelihood of IVF/ICSI success in patients with diminished ovarian reserve: a systematic review and meta-analysis. JBRA Assist Reprod. 2018;22(4):369-74.
2. Yilmaz N, Uygur D, Inal H, Gorkem U, Cicek N, Mollamahmutoglu L. Dehydroepiandrosterone supplementation improves predictive markers for diminished ovarian reserve: serum AMH, inhibin B and antral follicle count. Eur J Obstet Gynecol Reprod Biol. 2013;169(2):257-60.
3. Gebhardt KM, Feil DK, Dunning KR, Lane M, Russell DL. Human cumulus cell gene expression as a biomarker of pregnancy outcome after single embryo transfer. Fertil Steril. 2011;96(1):47-52.
4. Tsui KH, Lin LT, Horng HC, Chang R, Huang BS, Cheng JT. Gene expression of cumulus cells in women with poor ovarian response after dehydroepiandrosterone supplementation. Taiwan J Obstet Gynecol. 2014;53(4):559-65.

5. Yuan WS, Abu MA, Ahmad MF, Elias MH, Abdul Karim AK. Effects of Dehydroepiandrosterone (DHEA) Supplementation on Ovarian Cumulus Cells following In Vitro Fertilization (IVF)/Intra-Cytoplasmic Sperm Injection (ICSI) Treatment—A Systematic Review. Life (Basel). 2023;13(6):1237.
6. Lin LT, Wang PH, Wen ZH, Li CJ, Chen SN, Tsai EM, et al. The application of dehydroepiandrosterone on improving mitochondrial function and reducing apoptosis of cumulus cells in poor ovarian responders. Int J Med Sci. 2017; 14(6):585-94.
7. Lin LT, Cheng JT, Wang PH, Li CJ, Tsui KH. Dehydroepiandrosterone as a potential agent to slow down ovarian aging. J Obstet Gynaecol Res. 2017; 43(12):1855-62.
8. Neves AR, Montoya-Botero P, Polyzos NP. The Role of Androgen Supplementation in Women With Diminished Ovarian Reserve: Time to Randomize, Not Meta-Analyze. Front Endocrinol (Lausanne). 2021;12:653857.
9. Ferraretti AP, La Marca A, Fauser BC, Tarlatzis B, Nargund G, Gianaroli L; ESHRE working group on Poor Ovarian Response Definition. ESHRE consensus on the definition of 'poor response' to ovarian stimulation for in vitro fertilization: the Bologna criteria. Hum Reprod. 2011;26(7):1616-24.
10. Zhang Y, Zhang C, Shu J, Guo J, Chang HM, Leung PCK, et al. Adjuvant treatment strategies in ovarian stimulation for poor responders undergoing IVF: a systematic review and network meta-analysis. Hum Reprod Update. 2020;26(2):247-63.
11. Ovarian Stimulation TEGGO, Bosch E, Broer S, Griesinger G, Grynberg M, Humaidan P, et al. ESHRE guideline: ovarian stimulation for IVF/ICSI. Hum Reprod Open. 2020;2020(2):hoaa009.
12. ClinicalTrials.gov. (2023). Testosterone TRANSdermal Gel for Poor Ovarian Responders Trial (T-TRANSPORT). [online] Available from http://clinicaltrials.gov/ct2/show/NCT02418572 [Last accessed August, 2023].

CHAPTER 5

Dienogest

Kuldeep Jain, Maansi Jain

■ BACKGROUND

Dienogest is an orally active, synthetic, fourth-generation progestin, having a potent progestogenic and antiandrogenic and poor glucocorticoid activity. It has combined advantages of 19-nortestosterone and progesterone derivatives with minimal side effects. Its efficacy and safety are well researched and proven in clinical settings by various researchers. Its use is highly recommended to reduce endometriosis-associated pelvic pain (EAPP) in adolescent endometriosis as well as in reproductive age group.

■ CHEMICAL STRUCTURE

The chemical structure of dienogest is shown in **Figure 1**.

■ MECHANISM OF ACTION

Dienogest has both central and peripheral actions; thus, it provides the best clinical outcome.
- *Central effects:* It centrally acts on the hypothalamopituitary axis which leads to:
    - Inhibition of gonadotropin secretion: Moderate suppression of circulating estradiol and suppression of ovarian function resulting in an anovulatory cycle.

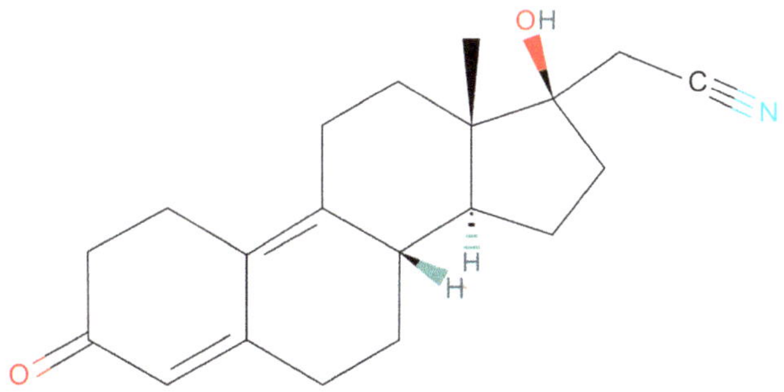

Fig. 1: Chemical structure of dienogest.

- *Local effects:* It exerts the following effects:
  - Antiproliferative
  - Anti-inflammatory
  - Antiangiogenic.

Dienogest by its action leads to an increase in matrix metalloproteinases, suppression of growth factors [epidermal growth factor (EGF), VGF, etc.], and decreased inflammatory reaction and peripheral estrogen, thus resulting in regression of endometriosis and pain relief.

■ SIDE EFFECTS

Dienogest is by and large well tolerated. Most common side effects are headache, breast discomfort, acne, nausea, vomiting, and weight gain. Some patients may also complain of depression and extreme flatulence. In a large, pooled study for an average duration of 39.8 weeks and maximum duration of up to 65 weeks, dienogest was given in doses of 2 mg continuously and was found to be well tolerated and efficacious in significant pain reduction.

■ DOSAGE AND EFFICACY

The usual dose of dienogest is 2 mg/day, and the drug can be given continuously or cyclically. Although it is effective, it is recommended to be given continuously for a prolonged period in order to be more effective. Dosage of 1 or 4 mg has been suggested which is used to improve the tolerability and increase the efficacy. In a phase II open level dose-finding study, dienogest was used in 1-, 2-, and 4-mg dosage for 24 weeks. The study concluded that the 2-mg dose was better tolerated with minimal side effects and was as efficacious as 4 mg in reducing the progression, pain, and recurrence rates. In another comparative double-blind placebo-controlled phase III trial, 2-mg dienogest was found to be well tolerated and superior to placebo in reducing EAPP with minimal adverse reaction. In another study, the visual analog scale (VAS) score was significantly lower with the dienogest group when used for 12 months.[1]

Dienogest has been studied for a prolonged period of 53 weeks continuously in a phase III trial for efficacy and recurrence of symptoms and was found to be well tolerated; the effect persisted for more than 2 years.[2] When compared to leuprolide acetate 3.75 mg for 3 months, dienogest showed equal efficacy (97% and 96%), lower frequency of hot flushes, and no change in bone mineral density (BMD) even at the end of 24-month therapy **(Fig. 2)**. These findings are reassuring for prolonged use of drug.[3]

Dienogest can also be used in abnormal uterine bleeding (AUB) associated with endometriosis in conjunction with leuprolide as a maintenance therapy. It decreases the total blood loss as well as episodes of break through bleeding.[4]

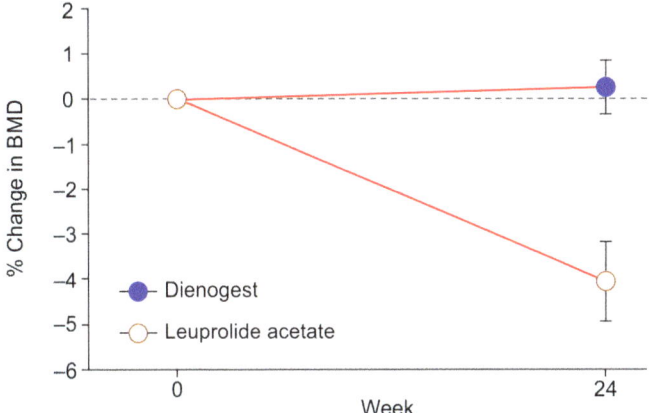

Fig. 2: Comparison between leuprolide acetate and dienogest regarding percentage change in bone mineral density (BMD).

■ CONCLUSION

Dienogest is an orally active, new-generation progestin with combined advantages of 19-nortestosterone and progesterone derivatives and is a highly effective, well-tolerable drug suitable for long-term use. There are no androgenic effects and minimal hypoestrogenic side effects.

■ REFERENCES

1. Strowitzki T, Faustmann T, Gerlinger C, Seitz C. Dienogest in the treatment of endometriosis-associated pelvic pain: a 12-week, randomized, double-blind, placebo-controlled study. Eur J Obstet Gynecol Reprod Biol. 2010;151(2):193-8.
2. Petraglia F, Hornung D, Seitz C, Faustmann T, Gerlinger C, Luisi S, et al. Reduced pelvic pain in women with endometriosis: efficacy of long-term dienogest treatment. Arch Gynecol Obstet. 2012;285(1):167-73.
3. Strowitzki T, Marr J, Gerlinger C, Faustmann T, Seitz C. Dienogest is as effective as leuprolide acetate in treating the painful symptoms of endometriosis: a 24-week, randomized, multicentre, open-label trial. Hum Reprod. 2010;25(3):633-41.
4. Kitawaki J, Kusuki I, Yamanaka K, Suganama I. Maintenance therapy with dienogest following gonadotropin-releasing hormone agonist treatment for endometriosis-associated pelvic pain. Eur J Obstet Gynecol Reprod Biol. 2011;157(2):212-6.

CHAPTER 6

Lactobacillus spp.

Pratap Kumar Narayan, Anjali Suneel Mundkur

■ BACKGROUND

Lactobacillus is a gram-positive aerotolerant or microaerophilic anaerobic gram-positive nonspore-forming rod-shaped bacteria. They form significant components of the human and animal microbiological environment of various body sites like the digestive system and female genital system. They form something called biofilms on various surfaces of the system. These biofilms protect them from the invasion of harmful pathogens. There is a mutually beneficial relationship between the host and the *Lactobacillus*. The host provides the source of nutrients while these bacteria protect against invasion by harmful pathogens.

Microbiology:[1]
- Class: Bacilli
- Domain: Bacteria
- Family: Lactobacillaceae
- Genus: *Lactobacillus*
- Order: Lactobacillales
- Phylum: Bacillota.

■ TYPES

The species of *Lactobacillus* is classified into three major groups. The bacterial metabolism establishes this division.[2]

1. *Obligate homofermentative group:* These organisms ferment lactose, glucose, and other sugars to lactic acid. Examples include *Lactobacillus acidophilus* and *Lactobacillus salivarius*.
2. *Facultative heterofermentative group:* In specific circumstances or with certain substrates, ferment sugars to generate ethanol, lactic acid, carbon dioxide, and acetic acid. Examples include *L. casei* and *L. plantarum*.
3. *Obligatory heterofermentative group:* This group of bacteria invariably ferments sugars to produce ethanol, lactic acid, carbon dioxide, and acetic acid. Examples include *L. reuteri* and *L. fermentum*.

Lactobacilli colonize several areas in the body. The most familiar systems are the gastrointestinal (GI) tract and the female genital tract. There is a mutualistic relationship with the human body.

They help in digestion and protection from pathogens. In return, the human body provides accommodation and nutrients required for metabolism.[3]

■ LACTOBACILLI IN GASTROINTESTINAL TRACT

The GI mucosa is considered one of the most crucial barrier sites of the body where foreign antigens, microbes, and potential pathogenic organisms come into close contact with host's immunological system. The semipermeable barrier allows for the absorption of nutrients and immune sensing. There is restriction of the influx of potentially harmful antigens and microbes.

Four elements compose the GI barrier.
1. *The mucosal layer:* It contains secretory immunoglobulin A (sIgA) molecules and antimicrobial peptides.
2. The commensal microbiota
3. *The gut-associated lymphoid tissue (GALT):* This constitutes several populations of immune cells in various compartments along the GI tract.
4. The intestinal epithelial cell (IEC) monolayer

These factors work together to maintain intestinal barrier integrity and homeostasis. Hence GI microbiota has a vital role to play in maintaining gut homeostasis.[4]

Uses of lactobacilli: The production of fermented dairy, meat or vegetable foods, and sourdough bread uses lactobacilli. The live microorganisms are widely used as probiotics, when given in adequate amounts, confer a health advantage on the host.

Lactobacilli are permitted a "generally recognized as safe (GRAS)" status from the US Food and Drug Administration (USFDA) and a "qualified presumption of safety (QPS)" status from the European Food Safety Authority (EFSA), hence allowing their use in food manufacture relatively effortless. Due to their economic value, lactobacilli are highly researched compared to other bacterial genera and are well characterized in genomics. There have been many studies concerning interactions with humans in terms of both health and disease. These qualities make *Lactobacillus* species an ideal probiotic candidate.[2]

An efficacious probiotic must have the ability to sustain and survive in the GI tract. It should be able to resist the low pH of the stomach, lack antibiotic resistance genes, and has to provide clear benefit to the host.

Further research is on its way by isolating probiotic-derived biomolecules to increase probiotics' efficiency, efficacy, safety, and quality. They are termed postbiotics, paraprobiotics, and heat-killed probiotics.

Tyndallized probiotics are the metabolic or secreted products of the bacteria, nonviable microbial cells (intact or broken), or crude cells extracts. They mainly include secreted peptides, proteins, enzymes, bacteriocins, short-chain fatty acids (SCFAs), organic acids, and cell envelope components of bacteria as well as peptidoglycans, teichoic acids, cell surface proteins, and cell wall polysaccharides.[5]

A consensus statement released by the International Scientific Association for Probiotics and Prebiotics (ISAPP) defines postbiotics as a "preparation of inanimate microorganisms and their components that confers a health benefit on the host. Effective postbiotics must contain inactivated microbial cells or cell components, with or without metabolites that contribute to observed health benefits".

Postbiotics also have several benefits over probiotics:
- There is no risk of translocation from the gut lumen to blood among vulnerable humans.
- No risk of accession and transfer of antibiotic resistance genes.
- No risk of interference with normal gut colonization in newborns.
- The active molecules released from the disrupted inactivated cells permeate through the mucus layers and trigger the epithelial cells directly.
- Cell death by cell lysis can produce further more composite beneficial effects.
- It is easier to extract, standardize, transport, and store. The benefits of postbiotics may represent a much better alternative to live probiotics and would be likely substitution for them in future.[6]

As shown in **Figure 1**, the intake of probiotics enhances the intestinal barrier function by higher mucus production, activating the release of antimicrobial peptides, and generation of sIgA production, more tight junction integrity of IECs and favoring competitive resistance against pathogens such as for host colonization receptors. Lactobacilli also improve the intestinal barrier resistance to infecting pathogens by competing for binding sites on IECs, glycoproteins in the mucus layer, or the plasminogen of extracellular matrix.[7]

■ *LACTOBACILLUS* IN THE FEMALE GENITAL TRACT

The vaginal microbiome alters with age, but for most healthy women of reproductive age, *Lactobacillus* species are the leading vaginal bacteria. *Lactobacillus crispatus*, *Lactobacillus gasseri*, *Lactobacillus jensenii*, and *Lactobacillus iners* are the dominant strains.[8]

The concentration of local estrogen is a key factor determining the profile of vaginal microbiota. An elevated estrogen content can induce a thicker, stimulate proton secretion by vaginal epithelial cells, and hasten glycogen deposition in the vaginal epithelium.[9]

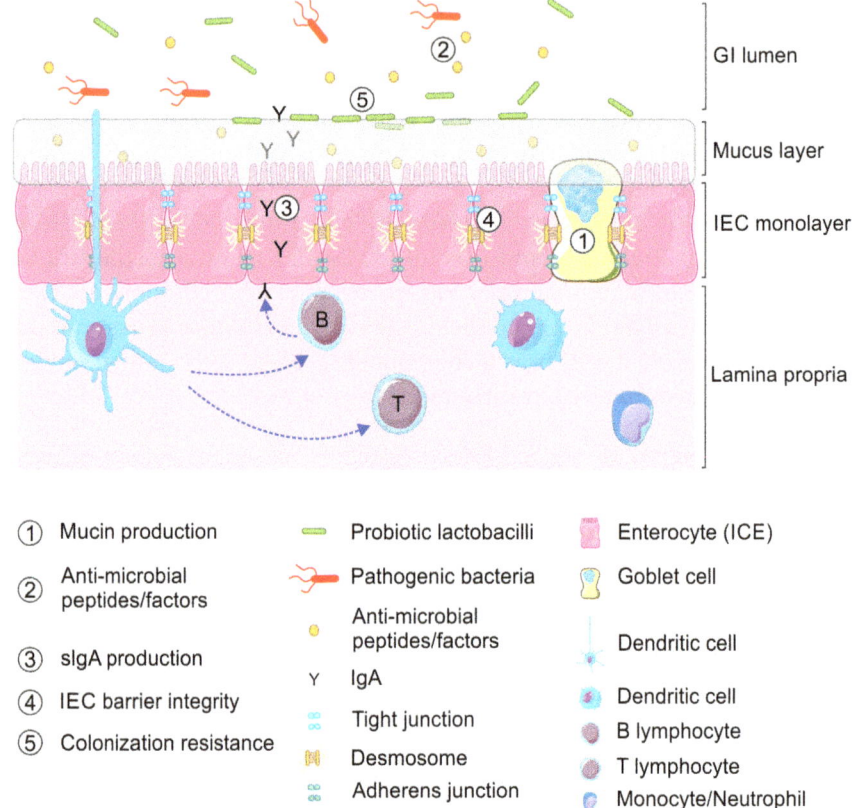

Fig. 1: Probiotic mechanisms of intestinal barrier enhancement.[2] (GI: gastrointestinal; IEC: intestinal epithelial cell; IgA: immunoglobulin A; sIgA: secretory immunoglobulin A)

■ LACTOBACILLI AS VAGINAL PROBIOTIC

The protective benefits of vaginal lactobacilli are ascribed to bactericidal factors, ecological niche, and immunomodulatory results.

Lactic acid produced by vaginal lactobacilli plays an important role. The benefits of lactic acid have been extensively studied. Research has shown that the physiological content of lactic acid in the vagina can successfully inactivate human immunodeficiency virus (HIV) and hamper the growth of uropathogenic and bacterial vaginosis (BV)-associated microbes. Deactivation of the pathogenic microbe is a significant effect; also, the immunomodulatory function plays a controversial role in this process.[10] Hydrogen peroxide (H_2O_2) is also a primary bactericidal material manufactured by vaginal *Lactobacillus* and lactic acid.[11]

The ability of acid production by the *Lactobacillus* species has become an important criterion when assessing their probiotic benefits. Based on an in vitro test, *L. crispatus* gathers a higher lactic acid accumulation compared with *L. iners*.[12] Hence, *L. crispatus* has a higher potency of probiotic effect than *L. iners*.

Vaginal *Lactobacillus* species *prevent the* incidence and development of cancer cells. In many studies, women with cervical intraepithelial neoplasia were likely to have low content of vaginal *Lactobacillus* species.[13] Inhibition of proliferation of the tumor cells has been studied.[14] It prevents infection by other organisms and reduces inflammation. This action of lactobacilli reduces the risk of cancer cervix and other gynecological cancers.[15]

Dysbiosis of vaginal microorganism frequently presents as bacterial vaginosis (BV). The vital characteristic of BV is the shift from a *Lactobacillus* predominant environment to a polymicrobial environment in the vagina.[16]

Bacterial vaginosis is a composite syndrome that is not caused by a particular organism. This nonspecific pathogenicity makes it hard to diagnose via a single criterion. The Nugent score and Amsel criteria are two often used standards to evaluate BV.[17]

The Nugent score focuses on the morphology of bacteria in vaginal smear, and Amsel criteria focus on the physical character of vaginal swab.

Bacterial vaginosis has an association with infertility. The ascending infection of BV associated microbes will hamper the function and immunity barrier of the upper genital tract.[18] Studies have shown the direct detrimental effect of BV-associated pathogens on ejaculated sperms. This gives an insight into the interaction between the vaginal microbiome and ejaculated spermatozoa.[19]

■ CLINICAL USES OF PROBIOTICS

Probiotics in diarrhea are:[20]
- *Traveler's diarrhea:* LGG = 2×10^9 CFU daily, start 2 days before departure and continue till return. *Saccharomyces boulardii* = $5 \times 10^{9-10}$ CFU daily, start 5 days before departure
- *Acute infectious diarrhea in infants and children:* LGG = 10^{10} CFU in 250 mL oral rehydration solution. *L. reuteri* = 10^{10-11} CFU daily for 5 days
- *Antibiotic-associated diarrhea:* LGG = 6×10^9 CFU daily for 1-4 weeks. *S. boulardii* = 4×10^9 CFU daily for 1-4 weeks. *L. acidophilus* and *Lactobacillus bulgaricus* = 2×10^9 CFU daily for 7 days
- *Clostridium difficile:* 2×10^{10} CFU daily for 4 weeks with vancomycin and metronidazole
- *Irritable bowel syndrome:* VSL# 3 = 9×10^{11} CFU daily for 8 weeks. *Bifidobacterium infantis* = 10^{6-10} CFU daily for 4 weeks. LGG = $8-9 \times 10^9$ CFU daily for 6 months.
- *Ulcerative colitis Crohn's disease: Escherichia coli* Nissle 1917 = 5×10^{10} CFU twice daily until remission. VSL # 3 = 8×10^{12} bacteria twice daily for 6 weeks with standard therapy. *Saccharomyces boulardii* = 250 mg 3 times daily for 4 weeks + mesalazine 1 g daily for 6 months.
- *Atopic dermatitis*

USES OF PROBIOTICS IN RESTORING REPRODUCTIVE HEALTH IN WOMEN[21]

- Restoration of normal vaginal flora and acidic pH
- When used in pregnant women, it helps to change from an anti-inflammatory to a proinflammatory state in the third trimester, which is required for labor. Reduces infantile eczema and allergy and reduced gestational diabetes mellitus, depression, and anxiety.
- Women with vaginal candidiasis—reduce vaginal candida load
- Improvement of vaginal microflora diversity, improving fertility rate
- Restoration of normal vaginal microenvironment in patients with BV.

SAFETY AND SIDE EFFECTS OF PROBIOTICS

The majority of probiotics are safe. However, care has to be taken when prescribing probiotics to severely ill or immunocompromised patients. There have been rare incidents of sepsis, endocarditis, and liver abscess during using *Lactobacillus*. Probiotics' most typical side effects are constipation, flatulence, hiccups, nausea, infection, and rash.

CONCLUSION

Lactobacillus is a gram-positive aerotolerant or microaerophilic anaerobic gram-positive nonspore-forming rod-shaped bacteria. Lactobacilli have colonized many areas in the human body, such as the GI tract and the female genital tract. An effective probiotic must have the capacity to sustain in the GI tract, resist the low pH of the stomach, lack antibiotic resistance genes, and has to benefit the host. The GI mucosa is the largest and one of the critical barrier sites of the body where microbes, foreign antigens, and potential pathogens come into contact with the host's immunological system. Use of probiotics can help treat many conditions related to skin and GI system and female and male reproductive system.

REFERENCES

1. Hammes WP, Hertel C. *Lactobacillus*. In: Whitman WB, Rainey F, Kämpfer P, Trujillo M, Chun J, DeVos P (Eds), et al. Bergey's Manual of Systematics of Archaea and Bacteria. Hoboken USA: John Wiley & Sons, Inc. (In Association with Bergey's Manual Trust); 2015. pp. 1-76.
2. Dempsey E, Corr SC. *Lactobacillus* spp. for gastrointestinal health: current and future perspectives. Front Immunol. 2022;6;13:840245.
3. Matos RC, Leulier F. Lactobacilli-Host Mutualism: "learning on the fly". Microb Cell Fact. 2014;13 (Suppl 1):S6.
4. Valenti P, Rosa L, Capobianco D, Lepanto MS, Schiavi E, Cutone A, et al. Role of lactobacilli and lactoferrin in the mucosal cervicovaginal defense. Front Immunol. 2018;9:376.

5. Nataraj BH, Ali SA, Behare PV, Yadav H. Postbiotics-parabiotics: the new horizons in microbial biotherapy and functional foods. Microb Cell Fact. 2020;19(1):168.
6. Teame T, Wang A, Xie M, Zhang Z, Yang Y, Ding Q, et al. Paraprobiotics and Postbiotics of Probiotic Lactobacilli, Their Positive Effects on the Host and Action Mechanisms: A Review. Front Nutr. 2020;7:570344.
7. Celebioglu HU, Svensson B. Dietary Nutrients, Proteomes, and Adhesion of Probiotic Lactobacilli to Mucin and Host Epithelial Cells. Microorganisms. 2018;6(3):90.
8. Nunn KL, Forney LJ. Unraveling the Dynamics of the Human Vaginal Microbiome. Yale J Biol Med. 2016;89(3):331-7.
9. Godha K, Tucker KM, Biehl C, Archer DF, Mirkin S. Human vaginal pH and microbiota: an update. Gynecol Endocrinol. 2018;34(6):451-5.
10. Witkin SS, Alvi S, Bongiovanni AM, Linhares IM, Ledger WJ. Lactic acid stimulates interleukin-23 production by peripheral blood mononuclear cells exposed to bacterial lipopolysaccharide. FEMS Immunol Med Microbiol. 2011;61(2):153-8.
11. Tachedjian G, O'Hanlon DE, Ravel J. The implausible "in vivo" role of hydrogen peroxide as an antimicrobial factor produced by vaginal microbiota. Microbiome. 2018;6(1):29.
12. Witkin SS, Mendes-Soares H, Linhares IM, Jayaram A, Ledger WJ, Forney LJ. Influence of vaginal bacteria and D- and L-lactic acid isomers on vaginal extracellular matrix metalloproteinase inducer: implications for protection against upper genital tract infections. MBio. 2013;4(4):e00460-13.
13. Mitra A, MacIntyre DA, Marchesi JR, Lee YS, Bennett PR, Kyrgiou M. The vaginal microbiota, human papillomavirus infection, and cervical intraepithelial neoplasia: what do we know and where are we going next? Microbiome. 2016;4(1):58.
14. Wang KD, Xu DJ, Wang BY, Yan DH, Lv Z, Su JR. Inhibitory Effect of Vaginal *Lactobacillus* Supernatants on Cervical Cancer Cells. Probiotics Antimicrob Proteins. 2018;10(2):236-42.
15. Ramchander NC, Crosbie EJ. The vaginal microbiome and gynecological cancer: exercise caution when considering causation. BJOG. 2018;125(3):316.
16. Onderdonk AB, Delaney ML, Fichorova RN. The Human Microbiome during Bacterial Vaginosis. Clin Microbiol Rev. 2016;29(2);223-38.
17. Kenyon CR, Osbak K. Recent progress in understanding the epidemiology of bacterial vaginosis. Curr Opin Obstet Gynecol. 2014;26(6):448-54.
18. Ravel J, Brotman RM. Translating the vaginal microbiome: gaps and challenges. Genome Med. 2016;8(1):35.
19. Zhang F, Dai J, Chen T. Role of *Lactobacillus* in Female Infertility Via Modulating Sperm Agglutination and Immobilization. Front Cell Infect Microbiol. 2021;10:620529.
20. Islam SU. Clinical uses of probiotics. Medicine. 2016;95(5).
21. Hashem NM, Gonzalez-Bulnes A. The Use of Probiotics for Management and Improvement of Reproductive Eubiosis and Function. Nutrients. 2022;14(4):902.

CHAPTER 7

Melatonin

Suchitra Pandit, Pratik Tambe

BACKGROUND

Infertility is a prevalent issue affecting millions of couples around the world. Infertility is a condition where a couple is unable to conceive a child despite several attempts. Various factors contribute to infertility including hormonal imbalances, poor ovulation, and sperm abnormalities. According to latest World Health Organization (WHO) data, 17.5% or one-sixth of all adults worldwide experience infertility. This is the result of a meta-analysis of 12,241 studies of which 133 were included in the final analysis.[1]

In recent years, the role of melatonin, a hormone primarily responsible for regulating sleep-wake cycles, has gained attention in the field of infertility. This article aims to explore the potential effects and mechanisms of melatonin on fertility as well as its applications in the treatment of infertility.

OVERVIEW OF MELATONIN

Melatonin is also known as the "sleep hormone" and is a naturally occurring hormone produced by the pineal gland in the brain **(Figs. 1 and 2)**. Its primary function is to regulate the sleep-wake cycle, helping maintain a sense of day and night. However, melatonin has now been discovered to have additional roles beyond sleep regulation. It is a potent antioxidant, scavenging harmful free radicals and protecting cells from oxidative stress. Additionally, melatonin is involved in the regulation of reproductive hormones and plays

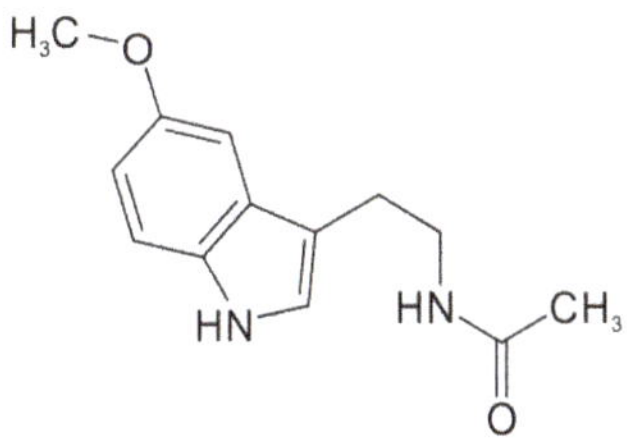

Fig. 1: Melatonin structure.

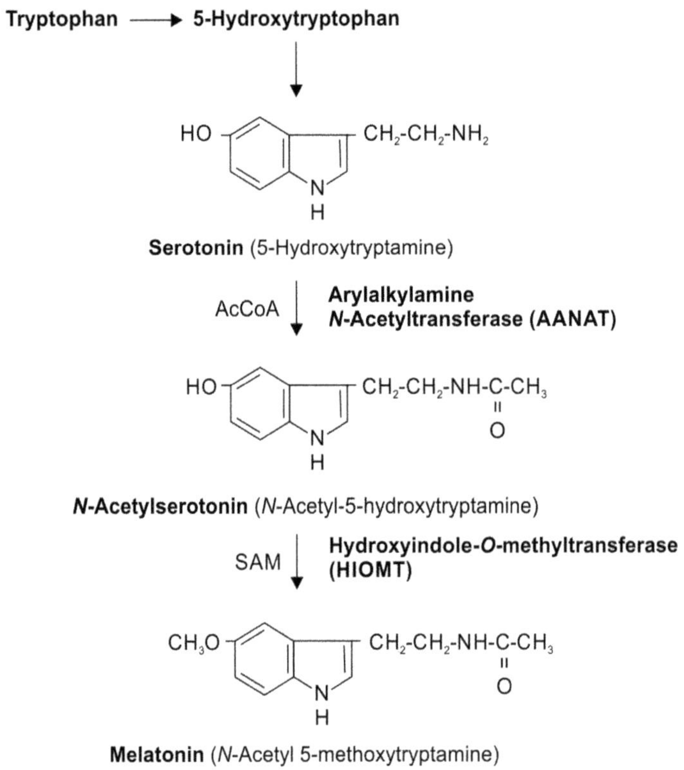

Fig. 2: Melatonin synthesis in the pineal gland.[2]

a crucial role in both female and male infertility. It should be noted that melatonin concentration dynamically changes within a day. In humans, melatonin secretion begins since nightfall, reaches a peak level in the middle of the night and decreases gradually during the second half of the night

Female Fertility

In women, melatonin acts directly on the ovaries exerting regulatory effects on the reproductive system. Studies have revealed that melatonin participates in the regulation of ovarian functions such as follicular growth and ovulation.

It has been found that women with fertility issues often have reduced melatonin levels. Low levels of melatonin can disrupt the menstrual cycle, impair ovulation, and increase the risk of miscarriage. Supplementing melatonin in women with infertility may provide promising results. In addition, melatonin has shown potential in protecting against oxidative stress-induced damage to the ovary, which is a key factor in female infertility.

Male Fertility

In men, maintenance of normal melatonin concentrations is essential and it has been linked to fertility. Melatonin receptors have been found in the testes, suggesting that melatonin may play a role in spermatogenesis. Oxidative stress is a significant factor in male infertility and the antioxidant properties of melatonin can help combat such oxidative stress. Several studies have demonstrated that melatonin supplementation improves semen quality, including sperm motility, morphology, and deoxyribonucleic acid (DNA) integrity. Furthermore, melatonin has been found to counteract the detrimental effects of environmental factors, such as electromagnetic radiation and toxins on male fertility.

■ LIFESTYLE FACTORS AND OXIDATIVE STRESS

Lifestyle factors, such as smoking, alcohol use, obesity, varicocele, infections, and psychological stress, which have been associated with infertility and poor sperm quality via the mechanisms of oxidative stress. This process is thought to influence 30–80% of infertile couples and hence, the category of male oxidative stress infertility (MOSI) was created. It has been suggested that increased oxidative activity may negatively impact the reproductive function by reducing sperm concentration, motility, and sperm DNA fragmentation.[3,4]

■ MELATONIN AND THE TESTIS

Melatonin has been found to regulate reproductive function via modulating the release of gonadotropin-releasing hormone (GnRH). Additionally, melatonin is absorbed by the testis, where it affects testicular function directly by acting on receptors present on Leydig, Sertoli, and intratesticular inflammatory cells. Interestingly, melatonin and testosterone both have comparable circadian rhythms and in animal species, the former influences various aspects of testicular function to facilitate seasonal reproduction.[5,6]

In particular, melatonin inhibits GnRH-induced testosterone release and stimulates the testicular conversion of testosterone into its active form dihydrotestosterone (DHT). This may occur via a local corticotropin-releasing hormone (CRH) system. Melatonin exerts antiproliferative and anti-inflammatory effects on testicular macrophages and mast cells. Its testicular concentrations show a negative correlation with concentrations of proapoptotic molecules and macrophages in infertile men.[7]

Melatonin functions as a free radical scavenger as noted above, preventing apoptosis and restoring testicular function. Exogenous administration of melatonin reduces the severity of induced testicular damage. It also acts on Sertoli cells, enhancing their responsiveness to follicle-stimulating hormone (FSH) and induces the secretion of growth factors active on spermatogonial stem cells proliferation.[8,9]

■ SCIENTIFIC EVIDENCE

A few clinical studies have investigated the impact of melatonin treatment on semen parameters. A possible correlation has been identified in both fertile and infertile men, categorizing the latter group by alterations in semen parameters. The authors observed lower melatonin levels in men affected by nonobstructive azoospermia, in those displaying impaired sperm motility and leukocytospermia (the levels of whom were lowest).[10]

In 2016, another group of researchers measured seminal plasma concentrations of melatonin and oxidative stress parameters in fertile normozoospermic and infertile teratozoospermic or azoospermic infertile men. The authors reported higher levels of seminal plasma melatonin in normozoospermic fertile men, with no difference between different subgroups of infertile men. Additionally, infertile men displayed increased concentrations of oxidation products in seminal fluid, with azoospermic patients displaying the highest levels. The study again highlights the possible relation between melatonin and oxidative stress in the infertile male.[11]

■ CLINICAL APPLICATION

Given the potential benefits of melatonin on fertility, researchers have started investigating its clinical applications in the treatment of infertility. Studies have shown that melatonin supplementation in infertile couples undergoing assisted reproductive techniques (ARTs) such as in vitro fertilization (IVF) may enhance pregnancy rates. Melatonin supplementation has been associated with improved oocyte quality, better embryo development, reduced miscarriage rates, and increased success rates during IVF treatment. However, more extensive studies are needed to establish the optimum dosage and duration of melatonin supplementation in infertility treatment.

A randomized control trial (RCT) published in 2018 highlighted the potential clinical benefit of melatonin supplementation on semen parameters after varicocele. Fifty-four infertile, mildly oligospermic men affected by varicocele were randomized to receive either 400 mg of melatonin or placebo after varicocele treatment. At the end of 3 and 6 months, the patients treated by melatonin showed a stronger improvement in terms of semen parameters (sperm concentration, motility, and proportions of normally formed spermatozoa), peripheral blood inhibin B levels, and total antioxidant compared with the placebo group.[12]

MELATONIN AND ASSISTED REPRODUCTIVE TECHNIQUES OUTCOMES

The role of melatonin on female reproduction has been extensively studied. Melatonin has been demonstrated to act on inflammation, apoptosis, and oxidative stress modulation as well.

Studies indicate that increased oxidative stress in the peritoneal, serum, and follicular microenvironments can result in poor oocyte quality in infertile women. Reducing the oxidative stress and reactive oxygen species in the microenvironment can protect the oocyte and the embryo. Recent studies have shown that melatonin concentration in the follicular fluid is associated with oocyte maturation rate and formation of good quality embryos in women undergoing IVF/ICSI (intracytoplasmic sperm injection).[13]

Hence, melatonin treatment in females for 3 mg per day or higher doses can significantly increase the serum and follicle concentration of melatonin. Researchers have therefore concluded that melatonin treatment can increase oocyte and embryo quality and subsequent pregnancy outcomes.[14]

In a systematic review and meta-analysis published 2020, the role of melatonin in ART has been elucidated. The authors concluded that melatonin is indeed associated with higher embryo quality and clinical pregnancy rate, but no significant improvement in live birth rates. Out of 116 articles, 10 studies matched the inclusion criteria. Clinical pregnancy was reported in all of the included studies and live birth was reported in three studies.

Melatonin treatment significantly increased the clinical pregnancy rate [odds ratio (OR) = 1.43 (1.11–1.86)] but not the live birth rate [(OR = 1.38 (0.78–2.46)]. Melatonin treatment increased the number of oocytes collected [standardized mean difference (SMD) = 0.34 (0.01–0.67)], the number of mature oocytes [SMD = 0.56 (0.27–0.85)], and the number of good quality embryos [mean difference (MD) = 0.36 (0.18–0.55)]. Melatonin treatment had no significant effect on the miscarriage rate [OR = 1.28 (0.65–2.51)].[15]

OVARIAN ANTIAGING

The mechanisms related to the antiovarian aging effects of melatonin are clearly not yet well defined. The clinical application of melatonin for the treatment of humans to improve ovarian physiology should have high priority in today's world when many women are delaying childbearing and suffering from infertility owing to ovarian aging. If long-term melatonin treatment prevents ovarian aging as represented by a decline in the number and quality of oocytes, they would have more oocytes of better quality when they undergo ART. Melatonin administration may therefore contribute to reproductive medicine to improve ART outcomes as there are currently no effective methods or established medications that prevent ovarian aging (**Figs. 3 to 5**).[16]

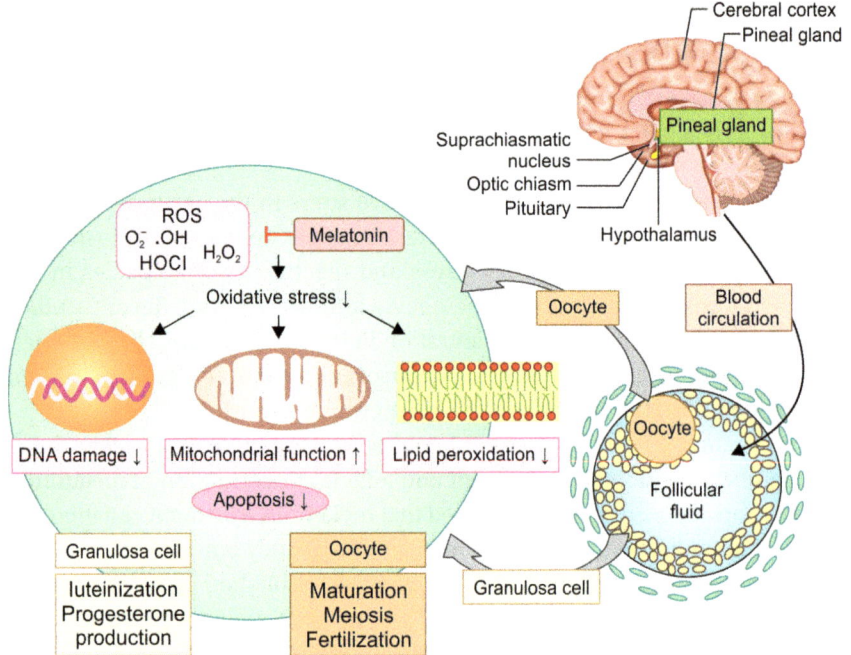

Fig. 3: Melatonin action on ovarian follicle.[16]

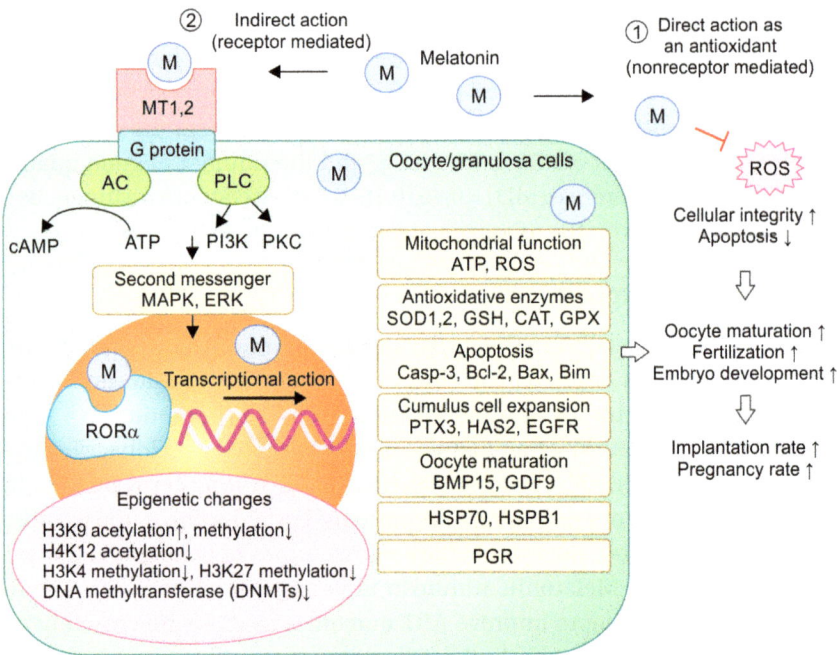

Fig. 4: Melatonin actions to improve oocyte quality.[16]

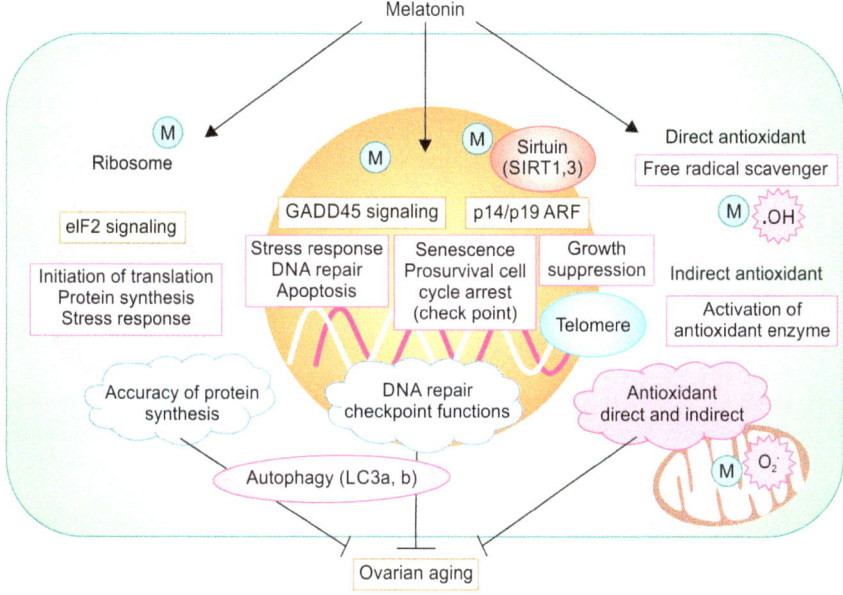

Fig. 5: Melatonin actions to prevent ovarian aging.[16]

■ CONCLUSION

Melatonin is important in the human body for regulating sleep-wake cycles. In addition, it appears to have significant implications in fertility, in both sexes. Its antioxidant properties and regulatory effects on the reproductive system suggest that melatonin plays a crucial role in maintaining and enhancing fertility. Melatonin supplementation in infertile couples has shown promising results, improving pregnancy rates, and enhancing the success of ARTs.

Melatonin administration significantly increases the clinical pregnancy rate in ART cycles. It also increases the number of oocytes collected, mature oocytes, and number of good quality embryos. There is no clear evidence that melatonin increases the adverse events in ART cycles. It has no significant effect on the live birth rate and these results need to be confirmed by future studies with a large sample size. Further research is also required to enhance our understanding of its mechanisms of action and its potential application as an adjunct therapy in infertility treatment.

■ REFERENCES

1. World Health Organization. (2023) Infertility. [online] Available from https://www.who.int/news-room/fact-sheets/detail/infertility [Last accessed August, 2023].

2. Arendt J, Aulinas A. Physiology of the Pineal Gland and Melatonin. In: Feingold KR, Anawalt B, Blackman MR, Boyce A, Chrousos G, Corpas E (Eds), et al. Endotext [Internet]. South Dartmouth (MA): MDText.com, Inc.; 2000.
3. Agarwal A, Parekh N, Panner Selvam MK, Henkel R, Shah R, Homa ST, et al. Male Oxidative Stress Infertility (MOSI): Proposed Terminology and Clinical Practice Guidelines for Management of Idiopathic Male Infertility. World J Mens Health. 2019;37(3):296-312.
4. Lucignani G, Jannello LMI, Fulgheri I, Silvani C, Turetti M, Gadda F, et al. Coenzyme Q10 and Melatonin for the Treatment of Male Infertility: A Narrative Review. Nutrients. 2022;14(21):4585.
5. Yang WC, Tang KQ, Fu CZ, Riaz H, Zhang Q, Zan LS. Melatonin regulates the development and function of bovine Sertoli cells via its receptors MT1 and MT2. Anim Reprod Sci. 2014;147:10-6.
6. Rossi SP, Windschuettl S, Matzkin ME, Terradas C, Ponzio R, Puigdomenech E. Melatonin in testes of infertile men: evidence for anti-proliferative and anti-oxidant effects on local macrophage and mast cell populations. Andrology. 2014;2:436-49.
7. Rocha CS, Martins AD, Rato L, Silva BM, Oliveira PF, Alves MG. Melatonin alters the glycolytic profile of Sertoli cells: implications for male fertility. Mol Hum Reprod. 2014;20:1067-76.
8. Chen C, Ling MY, Lin FH, Xu L, Lv ZM. Melatonin appears to protect against steroidogenic collapse in both mice fed with high-fat diet and H_2O_2-treated TM3 cells. Andrologia. 2019;51:e13323.
9. Deng SL, Wang ZP, Jin C, Kang XL, Batool A, Zhang Y, et al. Melatonin promotes sheep Leydig cell testosterone secretion in a co-culture with Sertoli cells. Theriogenology. 2018;106:170-7.
10. Awad H, Halawa F, Mostafa T, Atta H. Melatonin hormone profile in infertile males. Int J Androl. 2006;29:409-13.
11. Kratz EM, Piwowar A, Zeman M, Stebelová K, Thalhammer T. Decreased melatonin levels and increased levels of advanced oxidation protein products in the seminal plasma are related to male infertility. Reprod Fertil Dev. 2016;28:507-15.
12. Lu XL, Liu JJ, Li JT, Yang QA, Zhang JM. Melatonin therapy adds extra benefit to varicecelectomy in terms of sperm parameters, hormonal profile and total antioxidant capacity: a placebo-controlled, double-blind trial. Andrologia. 2018;50:e13033.
13. Zheng M, Tong J, Li WP, Chen ZJ, Zhang C. Melatonin concentration in follicular fluid is correlated with antral follicle count (AFC) and *in vitro* fertilization (IVF) outcomes in women undergoing assisted reproductive technology (ART) procedures. Gynecol Endocrinol. 2018;34:446-50.
14. Espino J, Macedo M, Lozano G, Ortiz A, Rodriguez C, Rodriguez AB, et al. Impact of melatonin supplementation in women with unexplained infertility undergoing fertility treatment. Antioxidants. 2019;8:E338.
15. Hu KL, Ye X, Wang S, Zhang D. Melatonin application in assisted reproductive technology: a systematic review and meta-analysis of randomized trials. Front Endocrinol. 2020;11:160.
16. Tamura H, Jozaki M, Tanabe M, Shirafuta Y, Mihara Y, Shinagawa M, et al. Importance of melatonin in assisted reproductive technology and ovarian aging. Int J Mol Sci. 2020;21(3):1135.

CHAPTER 8

New Generation Oral Contraceptive Pills

Neharika Malhotra, Umme Ruman

■ BACKGROUND

The oral contraceptive pill (OCP) is the most commonly used form of reversible contraception. The two types of OCPs are combined oral contraceptives (COCs), which contain estrogen and progesterone, and progestin-only pills (POPs). They have failure rates around 7.2–9% with typical use, and are safe for most patients. Estrogen-containing contraceptives specifically has the propensity to increase the risk of venous thromboembolism (VTE), patients with conditions associated with a risk of cardiovascular events better to avoid COCs.[1] The first OCP Enovid which was a combination of 10 μg of norethynodrel and 150 μg of mestranol, was approved by the Food and Drug Administration (FDA) in June 1960. In hormonal contraceptives, progestins are the most important agent that suppresses ovulation through their antigonadotropic properties.[2] To avoid the side effects caused by high estrogen content combined oral contraceptive pill (COCP), in 1960s and 1970s, "low dose" COC has been invented.[3] In the UK, the majority of COCP contain between 20 and 35 μg of the synthetic estrogen, ethinylestradiol (EE) instead of 50 μg. Both the components, estrogen and progesterone, have changed over time both in preparation and dose. All these changes are made to increase efficacy and safety profile and reduce side effects.

■ AIM

To know about the new oral contraceptive pills.

■ DISCUSSION

The primary mechanism of action of combined hormonal contraception (CHC) is prevention of ovulation. It acts on the hypothalamopituitary-ovarian axis to suppress luteinizing hormone (LH) and follicle-stimulating hormone (FSH) and thus inhibits ovulation.[4-7] Progesterone causes thickening of cervical mucus and alter tubal motility that may also contribute to the contraceptive effect.

■ CHANGE IN COMPONENTS
Estrogens
A COC product containing the synthetic estrogen, mestranol (metabolized to ethinylestradiol or EE) is available (50 µg mestranol roughly equates to 35 µg EE).[8] Now COC has been made available that contains 17β-estradiol. This is structurally identical to that which occurs naturally in humans. Safety profile of estradiol in COC could have improved compared to formulations containing EE or mestranol by reducing thrombotic and metabolic effects.[9] Although limited evidence suggests that estradiol COC is safe to use and highly effective in preventing unintended pregnancy,[10] yet further research will be required to assess the safety profile of estradiol COC relative to that of EE COC.

Progestogens
Progestogens are synthetic steroids possess some of the properties of progesterone. The advantages of synthetic progestogen are convenient dosing intervals, potent suppression of ovulation, and to prevent overproliferation of the endometrium in response to estrogen. Newer progestogens were developed to have fewer androgenic and glucocorticoid effects; some are antiandrogenic and have potentially favorable antimineralocorticoid effects.[11]

However, different progestogens may modify the effect of EE on hepatic clotting factors differently; CHC containing some newer progestogens in combination with EE appear to be associated with greater risk of VTE than COC containing other progestogens.

■ CATEGORIES OF PILL
The progestogens part of CHC are sometimes grouped by "generation", according to the time they were first marketed as constituents of COCs.[11,12] (Note that classification varies).
- *First:*
  - Estranes derived from testosterone include norethindrone, norethynodrel, norethindrone, acetate, and ethynodiol diacetate
  - Pregnanes derived from 17-OH progesterone include medroxy-progesterone acetate and chlormadinone acetate
- *Second:* Gonanes derived from testosterone include levonorgestrel and norgestrel
- *Third:* Gonane (levonorgestrel) derivatives include desogestrel, gestodene, norgestimate/norelgestromine, and etonogestrel norgestimate*
- *Newer/other:*
  - *Nonethylated estranes:* Dienogest and drospirenone
  - *Pregnanes (19-norprogesterones):* Nestorone, nomegestrol acetate, and trimegestone

(*Sometimes classified as second generation: LNG is one of its active metabolites).

Co-cyprindiol (containing 35 μg EE with cyproterone acetate, an antiandrogen) is indicated for management of moderate-to-severe acne and hirsutism. Women using co-cyprindiol for these indications do not require additional contraception.[13]

Fourth-generation Progesterone and Associated Risk of Venous Thromboembolism

Recently, drospirenone-containing oral contraceptives (OCs) which have a mineralocorticoid-derived progestational component are available. Gronich and colleagues[14] added further evidence of a higher relative risk of VTE among women taking this OC, in comparison to the alternatives of either third- or second-generation OCs. Dinger and colleagues carefully designed evaluations performed more recently have found evidence of such a risk.[15] The industry-funded phase IV European postmarketing surveillance study[14] collected data by mailed questionnaires from women who newly started COCP. In that study, all subgroups of pill users (categorized by additional risk factors or by drug prescribed) had a similar incidence of VTE, also excluded probability of higher incidence of thromboembolism by drospirenone. It also showed that efficacy of this progesterone-containing COCP is equal to other.[14] Subsequently, a large case–control study that evaluated a substantially larger database (in terms of women-years of pill use)[16] more convincingly demonstrated a difference in thrombotic risk. In these studies, authors compared incidence rates of idiopathic, nonfatal VTE between drospirenone users and levonorgestrel users, a comparison that emphasized the subset of events most likely influenced by the type of OC used. The increased risk ratio with drospirenone use remained significant across all age groups as well as with new and "switch" users.

Now according to hormonal activities, COCP can be categorized as follows:
- *Monophasic pills:* Monophasic OCPs contain a constant amount of estrogen and progestin in each active pill.[17]
  - Ethinylestradiol and norethindrone (Brevicon, Modicon, Wera, Balziva, and Briellyn, Gildagia, Philith, Zenchent)
  - Ethinylestradiol and norgestimate (Estarylla, Previfem, and Sprintec)
  - Drospirenone and ethinylestradiol (Ocella, Yasmin, Zarah, and Yaz)
  - Drospirenone, ethinylestradiol, and levomefolate (Safyral and Beyaz)
  - Ethinylestradiol and norgestrel (Cryselle, Elinest, and Ogestrel)
  - Ethinylestradiol and desogestrel (Apri, Desogen, Juleber, Reclipsen, and Solia)
  - Ethinylestradiol and levonorgestrel (Levora, Altavera, Daysee, Lessina, and Lybrel)
  - Ethinylestradiol and levonorgestrel extended-cycle (Amethia and Jolessa)
  - Estetrol/drospirenone (Nextstellis)

- *Biphasic pills:* Biphasic OCPs deliver the same amount of estrogen each day while progestin dose is increased halfway through cycle.
  - Ethinylestradiol and levonorgestrel extended-cycle (Amethia Lo, Camrese Lo, and Daysee)
  - Ethinylestradiol and desogestrel (Azurette, Kariva, Mircette, and Viorele)
  - Ethinylestradiol and levonorgestrel (LoSeasonique)
- *Triphasic pills:* Triphasic OCPs have three different doses of progestin and estrogen that change approximately every 7 days.
  - Ethinylestradiol and norethindrone (Aranelle, Tri-Norinyl, Leena, Alyacen 7/7/7, Necon 7/7/7, Notrel 7/7/7, Dasetta 7/7/7, and Cyclafem 7/7/7)
  - Ethinylestradiol and levonorgestrel (Enpresse and Trivora)
  - Ethinylestradiol and desogestrel (Caziant, Cyclessa, and Velivet)
  - Ethinylestradiol and norgestimate (TriNessa)
- *Four-phasic pills:* Four-phasic OCPs provide four different doses of progestin/estrogen during a 28-day cycle.
  - Dienogest and estradiol (Natazia)
  - Ethinylestradiol and levonorgestrel extended-cycle (Quartette)
- *Ninety-one-day pills:* Ninety-one-day OCPs provide a constant dose of estrogen and progestin for 84 days.
  - Ethinylestradiol and levonorgestrel (Introvale)
  - Ethinylestradiol and levonorgestrel extended-cycle (Amethia, Ashlyna, Jolessa, and Quasense)
  - Ethinylestradiol and levonorgestrel (Seasonique)
- *Progesterone-only pills:* Progesterone-only OCPs provide a constant dose of progestin.
  - Norethindrone (Aygestin, Camila, Errin, Jolivette, Lyza, Nora-BE, Nor-QD, and Ortho Micronor)

■ NEWER COMBINED ORAL CONTRACEPTIVE PILL

The US FDA has approved Nextstellis, a new OC that combines a novel estrogen, estetrol, with the well-known progestin drospirenone on April 16, 2021. The new OC contains 14.2 mg of estetrol and 3 mg of drospirenone.

Almost all currently prescribed OCs are formulated with ethinylestradiol, a synthetic and highly potent estrogen. Estetrol is naturally occurring, in contrast to ethinylestradiol and is produced from a plant source. An earlier clinical trial[18] found that an OC containing estetrol and drospirenone had substantially less impact on coagulation markers than an ethinylestradiol-drospirenone or an ethinylestradiol-levonorgestrel OC.

Recent phase 3 clinical trials conducted in North America and in Europe have found that the estetrol-drospirenone combination OC has contraceptive efficacy comparable with that of current OCs and is well tolerated, having a bleeding profile similar to familiar, current OCs. In the phase 3 trials, the new estetrol-drospirenone OC had minimal impact on triglyceride, cholesterol, or glucose levels.

When prescribed to appropriate candidates, OCs are a safe contraceptive option for millions of women. The main safety concern with combination estrogen-progestin OC use relates to a higher risk for VTE, which underscores the importance of not prescribing combination estrogen-progestin OCs, patches, or rings to women at elevated baseline VTE risk.

It is possible that this new estetrol-drospirenone OC is less likely to increase VTE risk than are conventional OCs formulated with ethinylestradiol. VTEs are uncommon events in OC users; thus, the potential safety advantage of this new estetrol-drospirenone pill over older formulations will not become clear until postmarketing epidemiologic studies can compare VTE risk with the estetrol OC versus an ethinylestradiol OC in large populations of women.

Ormeloxifene

Ormeloxifene is best known as a nonhormonal, nonsteroidal OC taken once a week. Available since the 1990s, it is marketed as centchroman.[19] When it was used as a contraceptive, there was improvement in menorrhagia and endometriosis, which led to control trials for the management of menorrhagia after its approval for this indication. In addition, it also reduced premenstrual symptoms, mastalgia, and dysmenorrhea by regularizing expression of estrogen receptors (ERs) on the endometrium, and it normalizes the bleeding from uterine cavity.

■ NEWER PROGESTERONE-ONLY PILL[20]

Levonorgestrel and Norethindrone

Levonorgestrel- and norethindrone-only progestins incompletely inhibit ovulation at the usual dosages (with individual components); the contraceptive effect is mainly due to the cervical mucus becoming impenetrable to sperm. An additional action of these POPs is their effect on the endometrium by desynchronizing ovulation and endometrial transformation in preparation for implantation. These preparations should be taken at the same time every day when used for regular contraception. The Pearl Index for typical use is between 6 and 8.

Desogestrel

The newer 75 µg desogestrel/day POP is taken continuously without a break. It inhibits ovulation and is as effective as CHC. This POP may be used as an estrogen-free inhibitor of ovulation. No major health risks are known. Breast cancer, active liver disease, and benign and malignant liver tumors (except nodular hyperplasia) are contraindications to its use.

The 4-mg Drospirenone-only Pill

This new POP is composed of 4 mg nonmicronized drospirenone and is used in a 24/4 day intake regimen. This regimen was chosen to improve the bleeding profile, maintain plasma E_2 levels comparable to those of the early follicular phase of the menstrual cycle, and maintain efficacy even when a pill is missed because drospirenone has a half-life of 30–34 hour. Its clinical development was based on the medical need for an estrogen-free contraceptive with the following characteristics:

- Contraceptive effectiveness comparable to that of COCs
- Improvement of the bleeding profile in comparison with other estrogen-free formulations; therefore, a regimen of 24 consecutive days of active tablet intake, followed by 4 days of placebo, was established to induce scheduled bleedings and reduce unscheduled bleeding and/or spotting.
- *Wide safety window:* The new 4 mg drospirenone formulation has a 24-hour missed pill safety window. This is an advantage not only over existing POPs but also over almost all COCs.
- Favorable safety profile, especially low to very low cardiovascular risk, i.e., venous and arterial thromboembolic events that are classically associated with EE use.
- Advantage of antimineralocorticoid and antiandrogenic effects.
- Adherence and acceptability thanks to the suitability of its administration.

■ CONCLUSION

Biomarkers of contraceptive efficacy or adverse effects, how individuals or groups metabolize contraception, initiation around reproductive life events, or the end of other methods are only a few of the still-largely-unknown topics of contraceptive research. In summary, a lot of new contraceptives have been produced in recent years to solve problems with older forms of birth control and develop new techniques. However, there are still a lot of open questions in the field of contraceptive research. Beyond its own technological implications, contraceptive technology offers a significant chance for completely individualized care.

■ REFERENCES

1. Brown EJ, Deshmukh P, Antell K. Contraception Update: Oral Contraception. FP Essent. 2017;462:11-9.
2. Scott JA, Brenner PF, Kletzky OA, Mishell DR Jr. Factors affecting pituitary gonadotropin function in users of oral contraceptive steroids. Am J Obstet Gynecol. 1978;130(7):817-21.
3. Dragoman MV. The combined oral contraceptive pill; recent developments, risks and benefits. Best Pract Res Clin Obstet Gynaecol. 2014;28:825-34.
4. Cohen BL, Katz M. Pituitary and ovarian function in women receiving hormonal contraception. Contraception. 1979;20:475-87.

5. Cohen BL, Katz M. Further studies on pituitary and ovarian function in women receiving hormonal contraception. Contraception. 1981;24:159-72.
6. Crosignani PG, Testa G, Vegetti W, Parazzini F. Ovarian activity during regular oral contraceptive use. Contraception. 1996;54:271-3.
7. Mulders TM, Dieben TO. Use of the novel combined contraceptive vaginal ring NuvaRing for ovulation inhibition. Fertil Steril. 2001;75:865-70.
8. Christin-Maitre S. History of oral contraceptive drugs and their use worldwide. Best Pract Res Clin Endocrinol Metab. 2013;27:3-12.
9. Lete I, Chabbert-Buffet N, Jamin C, Lello S, Lobo P, Nappi RE, et al. Haemostatic and metabolic impact of estradiol pills and drospirenone-containing ethinylestradiol pills vs. levonorgestrel-containing ethinylestradiol pills: a literature review. Eur J Contracept Reprod Health Care. 2015;20:329-43.
10. Christin-Maitre S, Laroche E, Bricaire L. A new contraceptive pill containing 17β-estradiol and nomegestrol acetate. Womens Health (Lond). 2013;9:13-23.
11. Sitruk-Ware LR, Mishell DR (Eds). Progestins and antiprogestins in clinical practice. New York: Marcel-Dekker; 2000.
12. Schindler AE, Campagnoli C, Druckmann R, Huber J, Pasqualini JR, Schweppe KW, et al. Classification and pharmacology of progestins. Maturitas. 2003;46 (Suppl 1):S7-16.
13. Van Vliet HA, Grimes DA, Lopez LM, Schulz KF, Helmerhorst FM. Triphasic versus monophasic oral contraceptives for contraception. Cochrane Database Syst Rev. 2011;CD003553.
14. Gronich N, Lavi I, Rennert G. Higher risk of venous thrombosis associated with drospirenone-containing oral contraceptives: a population-based cohort study. CMAJ. 2011;183:2103.
15. Dinger JC, Heinemann LAJ, Kühl-Habich D. The safety of a drospirenone-containing oral contraceptive: final results from the European Active Surveillance Study on oral contraceptives based on 142475 women-years of observation. Contraception. 2007;75:344-54.
16. Jick SS, Hernandez RK. Risk of non-fatal venous thromboembolism in women using oral contraceptives containing drospirenone compared with women using oral contraceptives containing levonorgestrel: case-control study using United States claims data. BMJ. 2011;342:d2151.
17. Bennett PN, Brown MJ, Sharma P. Hypothalamic pituitary and sex hormones. Clinical Pharmacology, 11th edition. Philadelphia: Elsevier Ltd.; 2012. pp. 596-814.
18. Drugs.com (2021). Nextstellis FDA Approval History. https://www.drugs.com/history/nextstellis.html [Last accessed August, 2023].
19. Pati T, Chanania K, Marandi S, Hansa J. Ormeloxifene: Looking beyond contraception. J Midlife Health. 2017;8(1):17-20.
20. Palacios S, Regidor PA, Colli E, Skouby SO, Apter D, Roemer T, et al. Oestrogen-free oral contraception with a 4 mg drospirenone-only pill: new data and a review of the literature. Eur J Contracept Reprod Health Care. 2020;25(3):221-7.

CHAPTER 9

Parenteral Iron

PK Shah

■ BACKGROUND

Iron deficiency anemia (IDA) is the most common cause of anemia worldwide. This needs proper treatment. In underdeveloped or developing countries, estimates of the prevalence of iron deficiency have ranged from 30–70%.[1]

Iron deficient states may develop due to unmet increased metabolic iron requirement or inadequate supply state. Iron deficiency is associated with underlying conditions including chronic kidney disease, heart failure, underlying inflammatory conditions, cancer and bariatric surgery, menorrhagia, IDA in pregnancy, and postpartum bleeding.[2] Iron is not only the key driver for erythropoiesis and formation of red blood cells.[3] Iron is also a critical element in cellular processes.

■ STAGES OF IRON DEFICIENCY

Figure 1 depicts the stages of iron deficiency.

■ ORAL IRON THERAPY

In 19th century ferrous sulfate was introduced and became the standard treatment for IDA.[4] Oral iron supplementation is the first choice because

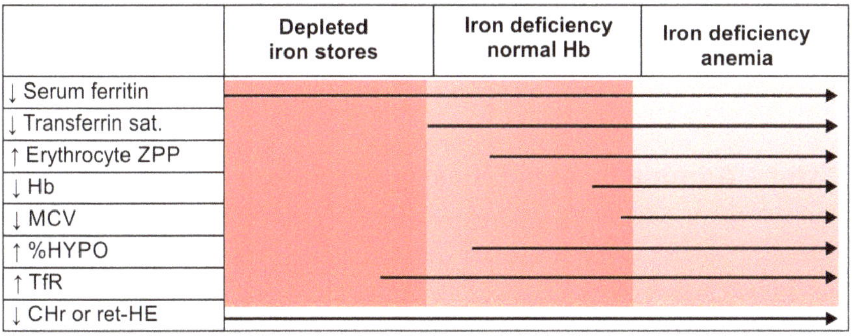

	Depleted iron stores	Iron deficiency normal Hb	Iron deficiency anemia
↓ Serum ferritin			
↓ Transferrin sat.			
↑ Erythrocyte ZPP			
↓ Hb			
↓ MCV			
↑ %HYPO			
↑ TfR			
↓ CHr or ret-HE			

Fig. 1: Alterations in biochemical and hematological parameters at various stages of iron deficiency. (CHr or ret-HE: reticulocyte hemoglobin content; Hb: hemoglobin; MCV: mean corpuscular volume; Transferrin sat.: serum transferrin saturation; ZPP: zinc protoporphyrin; TfR: serum transferrin receptor; %HYPO: %hypochromic erythrocytes)

treatment is simple, inexpensive, and relatively effective. In adults, the recommended daily dose range is 150-200 mg/day; for children 3-6 mg iron/kg body weight/day.

> *Causes of treatment failure in oral iron therapy:*
> - Lack of adherence to therapy or insufficient length of therapy
> - Concomitant/causal underlying blood loss pathology not resolved:
>   - Poor duodenal absorption
>   - Concomitant gastrointestinal (GI) pathology (inflammatory bowel disease or any other cause or chronic inflammation; malignancy)
>   - Insufficient gastric acidity (pharmacological blockade of gastric secretion)
> - Side effects:
>   - Nausea
>   - Constipation
>   - Upper GI irritation
>   - Black or dark green stools

In addition to this, in inflammatory bowel syndrome (IBD), the possibility that iron may further damage the intestinal mucosa should be a serious indication for the use of intravenous (IV) rather than oral iron therapy.[5,6]

■ INTRAVENOUS IRON

Treatment with IV iron is superior to oral iron and presents several advantages such as faster and higher increase in hemoglobin (Hb) levels and replenishment of body iron stores. The modern formulations of IV iron have emerged as safe and effective alternatives for IDA management.

> *Clinical indications for intravenous (IV) iron treatment:*
> - Cancer-related anemia
> - Postpartum iron deficiency anemia
> - Anemia of pregnancy
> - Anemia of chronic kidney disease
> - Anemia of inflammatory bowel disease
> - In iron malabsorption syndromes [postgastrectomy, Biermer's disease, iron-refractory iron deficiency anemia (IRIDA)]
> - Intolerance of or noncompliance with oral iron treatment

History, Administration, Efficacy, and Safety

The first salt introduced for parenteral early in the 20th century was *ferric hydroxide*. However, the lack of a carbohydrate shell resulted in immediate iron release and severe toxic reactions. Its use is currently restricted.[7]

Available Intravenous Iron Preparations

The first *high-molecular-weight iron dextran (HMW-ID)* for intramuscular (IM) and IV use (Imferon) was introduced in 1954.[8] HMW-ID is an iron oxyhydroxide core, surrounded by a carbohydrate shell made of polymers of dextran. The increased incidence of serious adverse events (AEs) reported. The well-known dextran-induced anaphylactic reactions led to its recommendation only in extreme clinical conditions.

In 1992, formulations containing *low-molecular-weight iron dextran (LMW-ID)* (INFeD, Cosmofer) were approved for clinical use. This can be administered as an IV bolus or total dose infusion (TDI) up to 1,000 mg. It required a test dose and had black box warnings.[7]

In 1999, *ferric gluconate (FG)* (Ferrlecit) was introduced. A historical review of the use of FG and iron dextrans concluded that FG was a safer therapeutic option and its safety was related to the lack of the dextran envelope and associated with a lower risk of anaphylactic reactions.[9,10]

In November 2000, *iron sucrose (IS)* (Venofer) was approved. IS is safely administered as a 15–30 minute infusion in doses of 200–300 mg; the maximum weekly dose should not exceed 600 mg. AEs are rarely observed.[11,12] The main disadvantage of IS is the need for multiple infusions.

Ferric carboxymaltose (FCM) is a new parenteral dextran-free iron product approved for rapid and high-dose replenishment of depleted iron stores. FCM is an iron complex that consists of a ferric hydroxide core stabilized by a carbohydrate shell. FCM allows controlled delivery of iron with minimal risk of releasing large amounts of ionic iron into the serum.[13]

Ferric carboxymaltose is a stable complex with a very low immunogenic potential. It permits the administration of large doses (15 mg/kg; maximum of 1,000 mg/infusion) in a single and rapid (15-minute) infusion without the requirement of a test dose.[14,15] But the risk is associated with higher incidences of hypophosphatemia, which leads to development of brittle bones.[16]

Iron isomaltoside 1000 (Inj I3) is the newest IV iron agent, which is a nonbranched, nonanaphylactic carbohydrate, structurally different from dextran. Iron isomaltoside has a very low immunogenic potential and a very low content of free iron and can therefore be administered as a rapid high-dose infusion of up to 2,000 mg without the application of a test dose. The structure is somehow different, as the linear oligosaccharide isomaltoside 1000 allows the formation of a matrix with interchanging iron and carbohydrate, instead of a classical spheroidal iron carbohydrate nanoparticle.[17]

The use of these stable compounds carries benefits for both the patient (less disruption of life, less time away from home/work, reduced injections, few side effects, etc.) and the hospital/health service (reduced visits, reduced physician and nurse time, improved outpatient management, improved cost-effectiveness, etc.). Other benefits of high-dose or three times daily (TID) infusions are the significant reduction of treatment period[17] and the higher serum ferritin levels obtained.[18]

Administration Specifics

The dosage calculation is done by the Ganzoni formula. It is administered by the IV route by infusion given in 100 mL normal saline over 15–20 minutes. After IV administration the iron (III)-Isomaltoside 1000 is rapidly taken up by the reticuloendothelial system (RES), particularly in the liver and spleen. From there the iron is slowly released.

■ INTRAMUSCULAR IRON PREPARATIONS

Iron sorbitex,[19] *iron dextran, and iron polymaltose* can be administered via the IM route. These formulations have significant beneficial results but limitations to use by the IM route like burning/pain, swelling, blackening at site of injection, nausea, vomiting, and giddiness observed in patients.[20] They were widely used previously, but due to their multiple side effects the use has declined gradually. The IM route has now been replaced by the IV route, which has now become the preferable route of choice for administration of parenteral iron.

■ HYPERSENSITIVITY REACTIONS

Intravenous iron is increasingly used for the treatment of IDA. While acute reactions during iron infusions are very infrequent, they can be life-threatening.

> *Guidance for risk management:*[21]
> - All intravenous (IV) iron preparations carry a small risk of adverse reactions, which can be life-threatening if not treated promptly.
> - IV iron products should be administered only when staff trained to evaluate and manage anaphylactic reactions, as well as resuscitation facilities are immediately available.
> - Patients should be closely monitored for signs of hypersensitivity during and for at least 30 minutes after each administration.
> - All IV iron products are contraindicated in patients with known serious hypersensitivity to any parenteral iron product.
> - IV iron should not be given to pregnant women in the first trimester. Careful risk/benefit evaluation is required before use in the second or third trimester.
> - Special precautions are needed if IV iron is to be given to patients with known allergies (including drug allergies), severe atopy, or systemic inflammatory diseases (e.g., systemic lupus erythematosus and rheumatoid arthritis).

Factors increasing risk and/or severity of hypersensitivity reactions (HSRs) in patients given iron infusion are:
- Previous reaction to IV iron
- Fast iron infusion rate
- History of other drug allergy or allergies
- Severe asthma or eczema

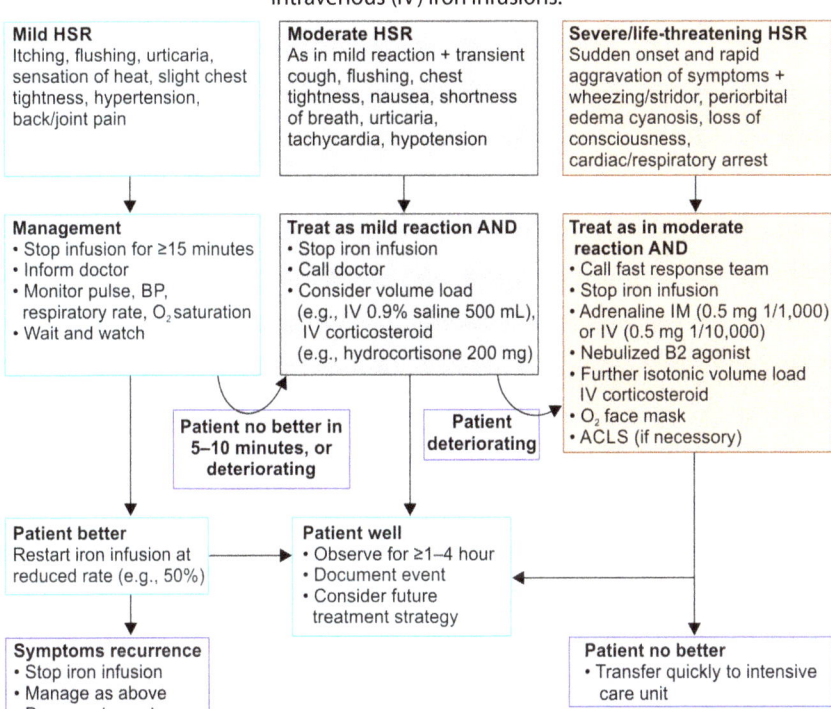

Flowchart 1: Grading and management of acute hypersensitivity reactions (HSRs) to intravenous (IV) iron infusions.

(ACLS: advanced cardiovascular life support; BP: blood pressure; IM: intramuscular)

- Mastocytosis
- Severe respiratory or cardiac disease
- Old age
- Treatment with beta blockers, angiotensin-converting enzyme (ACE) inhibitors
- First trimester of pregnancy—IV iron is contraindicated in early pregnancy
- Systemic inflammatory disease (e.g., rheumatoid arthritis and lupus erythematosus) **(Flowchart 1).**

CONCLUSION

Iron deficiency is the most common cause of anemia worldwide. In the great majority of cases oral iron therapy represents an effective, inexpensive, and safe way of treating this pathologic entity. There are however some specific situations where because of decreased or abolished duodenal iron absorption parenteral iron administration is mandatory.

In the past IV iron preparations were considered dangerous because of the risk of life-threatening allergic reactions. The introduction of new iron–carbohydrate complexes has eliminated this danger. As the organism possesses no mechanism for eliminating iron, when giving an IV iron preparation, we must always calculate total iron needs to avoid iron toxicity secondary to iron overload.

■ REFERENCES

1. Brittenham G. Disorders of iron metabolism: iron deficiency and iron overload. In: Hoffman R, Benz EJ, Shattil SJ, Furie B, Silberstein LE, McGlave P (Eds). Hematology: Basic Principles and Practice. Philadelphia: Churchill Livingstone Elsevier, 2009. pp. 453-74.
2. Macdougall IC, Comin-Colet J, Breymann C, Spahn DR, Koutroubakis IE. Iron sucrose: a wealth of experience in treating iron deficiency. Adv Ther. 2020;37:1960-2002.
3. Richards T, Breymann C, Brookes MJ, Lindgren S, Macdougall IC, McMahon LP, et al. Questions and answers on iron deficiency treatment selection and the use of intravenous iron in routine clinical practice. Ann Med. 2021;53(1):274-85.
4. Blaud P. Sur les maladies chloropiques et sur un mode de traitement specifique dons ces affecions]. Rev Med Fr Etrang. 1832;45:357-67 French.
5. Muñoz M, Gómez-Ramírez S, García-Erce JA. Intravenous Iron in inflammatory bowell disease. World J Gastroenterol. 2009;15(37):4666-74.
6. Lindgren S, Wikman O, Befrits R, Blom H, Eriksson A, Granno C, et al. Intravenous iron sucrose is superior to oral iron sulphate for correcting anaemia and restoring iron stores in IBD patients: a randomized, controlled, evaluator-blind, multicentre study. Scand J Gastroenterol. 2009;44(7):838-45.
7. Auerbach M, Ballard H. Clinical use of intravenous iron: administration, efficacy and safety. Am Soc Hematol Educ Program. 2010;338-47.
8. Fishbane S, Kowalski EA. The comparative safety of intravenous iron dextran, iron saccharate, and sodium ferric gluconate. Semin Dial. 2000;13(6):381-4.
9. Faich G, Strobos J. Sodium ferric gluconate complex in sucrose; safer intravenous iron therapy than iron dextrans. Am J Kidney Dis. 1999;33(3):464-70. Comment in: Am J Kidney Dis. 1999;33(3):595-7.
10. Panesar A, Agarwal R. Safety and efficacy of sodium ferric gluconate complex in patients with chronic kidney disease. Am J Kidney Dis. 2002;40(5):924-31.
11. Aronoff GR, Bennett WM, Blumenthal S, Charytan C, Pennell JP, Reed J, et al.; United States Iron Sucrose (Venofer) Clinical Trials Group. Iron sucrose in hemodialysis patients: safety of replacement and maintenance regimens. Kidney Int. 2004;66(3):1193-8.
12. Chaytan C, Schwenk MH, Al-saloum MM, Spinowitz BS. Safety of iron sucrose in hemodialysis patients intolerant to other parenteral iron products. Nephron Clin Pract. 2004;96(2):c63-6.
13. Lyseng-Williamsom KA, Keating GM. Ferric carboxymaltose. A review of its use in iron-deficiency anaemia. Drugs. 2009;69(6):739-56.
14. Kulnigg S, Stoinov S, Simanenkov, Dudar LV, Karnafel W, Garcia LC, et al. A novel intravenous iron formulation for treatment of anemia in inflammatory bowel disease: the ferric carboxymaltose (FERINJECT) randomized controlled trial. Am J Gastroenterol. 2008;103(5):1182-92.

15. Covic A, Mircescu G. The safety and efficacy of intravenous iron carboxymaltose in anaemic patients underoing haemodialysis: a multi-centre, open-label, clinical study. Nephrol Dial Trans. 2010;25(8):2722-30.
16. Wolf M, Rubin J, Achebe M, Econs MJ, Peacock M, Imel EA, et al. Effects of Iron Isomaltoside vs Ferric Carboxymaltose on Hypophosphatemia in Iron-Deficiency Anemia. JAMA. 2020;323(5):432-43.
17. Jahn MR, Andreasen HB, Futterer SA, Nawroth T, Schunemann V, Kolb U, et al. A comparative study of the physicochemical properties of iron isomaltoside 1000 (Monofer), a new intravenous iron preparation and its clinical implications. Eur J Pharm Biopharm. 2011;78(3):480-91.
18. FDA. (2021). Monofer Prescribing Information Switzerland. [online] Available from: https://www.accessdata.fda.gov/drugsatfda_docs/label/2020/208171s000lbl.pdf [Last accessed August, 2023].
19. USP 39 page no. 4396.
20. Dhanani JV, Ganguly BP, Chauhan LN. Comparison of efficacy and safety of two parenteral iron preparations in pregnant women. J Pharmacol Pharmacother. 2012;3(4):314-9.
21. Rampton D, Folkersen J, Fishbane S, Hedenus M, Howaldt S, Locatelli F, et al. Hypersensitivity reactions to intravenous iron: guidance for risk minimization and management. Haematologica. 2014;99(11).

CHAPTER 10

Berberine

Pratik Tambe

■ BACKGROUND

Of late, there has been a growing interest in natural remedies, herbal medicine and lifestyle management, which has grown significantly. Among these, berberine is a compound that has attracted widespread attention among lay persons interested in health and fitness as well as medical practitioners and researchers. Berberine is a bioactive alkaloid isolated from plants of the genus *Berberis*, including *Berberis vulgaris*, *Berberis aristata*, *Hydrastis canadensis*, *Coptis japonica,* and *Coptis chinensis*. It is primarily found in the roots, rhizomes, and stems of these plants.[1]

■ HISTORY

Berberine has a long history of usage in traditional Chinese and Ayurvedic medicine. It has been commonly prescribed to treat diarrhea and combat infections. It also has a role to play in enhancing cardiovascular health and for regulating blood sugar levels. Hence, it has generated immense interest as researchers investigate in modern fashion the scientific basis behind these ancient remedies and explore their application and place in the modern clinician's armamentarium **(Fig. 1)**.

■ MECHANISM OF ACTION

Ongoing research has highlighted several mechanisms whereby berberine exerts its action. One of its primary actions is activating an enzyme called AMP-activated protein kinase (AMPK) which plays a crucial role in regulating

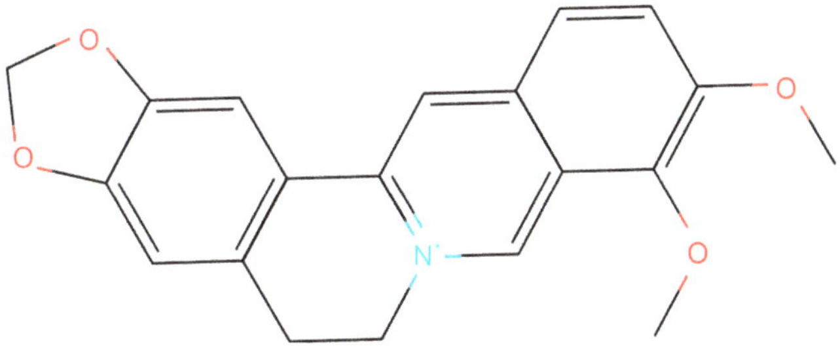

Fig. 1: Chemical structure of berberine.[1]

cellular energy metabolism, promoting insulin sensitivity and reducing inflammation. Therefore, by enhancing AMPK activation at a cellular level, berberine has the potential to stimulate glucose uptake and improve blood sugar control.

Berberine has also been found to impact various cellular signaling pathways which are associated with lipid metabolism. It inhibits the activity of an enzyme called PCSK9 (proprotein convertase subtilisin/kexin type 9), leading to increased clearance of low-density lipoprotein (LDL) cholesterol from the bloodstream. In addition, berberine activates a protein called farnesoid X receptor (FXR), which regulates the expression of genes involved in cholesterol synthesis and bile acid metabolism.

Fifteen potential targets of berberine, e.g., aldo-keto reductase family 1 member C3 (AKR1C3), insulin receptor, estrogen receptor, and tyrosine-protein phosphatase nonreceptor type 1 have been found. Therefore, it is quite clear that the action of berberine on human physiology is multipronged and varied. It acts on various metabolic processes and may thus have immense potential in impacting a number of biochemical pathways in the human body.[2]

▪ INSULIN RESISTANCE

Berberine activates the insulin signaling pathways, as per recent research. It has been found that in diabetic mice treated with berberine, hyperglycemia was reduced and the impaired glucose tolerance was improved, but insulin release or synthesis was not increased. This effect is mediated via its ability to inhibit the catalysis of protein tyrosine phosphatase 1B (PTP1B) and enhance the phosphorylation of insulin receptor and insulin receptor substrate-1 (IRS1) in 3T3-L1 adipocytes.[3]

Berberine is responsible for regulating the IRS1 signaling pathway. It also activates the expression of key proteins in PI3K/Akt/GSK-3β insulin signaling pathway and increases the phosphorylation of Akt. It inhibits mitogen-activated protein kinase (MAPK) pathway, a critical signal transduction pathway, which leads to an inseparable link between androgen biosynthesis and IR. It can increase the expression of peroxisome proliferator activated receptors (PPARs) α and γ in endometrium, and improve impaired glucose tolerance.[4,5]

Berberine promotes the transport and consumption of glucose in adipocytes and inhibits the differentiation of adipocytes. Oxygen-dependent glucose oxidation was inhibited and glycolysis was enhanced in polycystic ovary syndrome (PCOS) obese women on berberine. It enhances ubiquitination of Sirtuin 3 (SIRT3), a major mitochondria nicotinamide adenine dinucleotide (NAD+)-dependent deacetylase, and then leads to AMP accumulation, which can activate AMPK signaling and further promotes glucose uptake. Berberine promotes glucose uptake and upregulates the expression of Glut4 in the ovary. This is its primary mechanism behind reducing the harmful effects of PCOS and insulin resistance (IR).[6,7]

■ ANDROGEN LEVELS

Berberine has been shown to reduce androgen levels. This effect is mediated via a variety of mechanisms including increased sex hormone-binding globulin (SHBG) levels peripherally and expression of SHBG in the endometrial stroma. It also suppresses androgen receptor signaling pathways by inducing protein degradation instead of receptor activation and messenger RNA (mRNA) expression. AMPK-α is phosphorylated at Ser485/491 by Akt, thus making it difficult for AMPKα to be phosphorylated at Thr172, which reduces the activity of AMPK.[8,9]

Berberine reduces serum testosterone levels by reducing the density of steroidogenetic acute regulatory protein (StAR) on the cell membrane of follicular membrane cells. StAR promotes the cholesterol transport from outside the mitochondrial membrane to the inner membrane and is a key step in the production of androgens by theca cells. It also suppresses aldo-keto reductase 1C3 (AKR1C3) activity, which catalyzes the conversion of low active hormone precursors such as androstenedione and androsterone to highly active testosterone and dihydrotestosterone in the last two steps of steroid synthesis.

It also downregulates the expression of *CYP17a1* gene in ovary and upregulates the expression of *CYP19a1* in the ovary. *CYP17a1* encodes the steroid-producing enzyme cytochrome p45017 α-hydroxylase (P450c17), which is required for the synthesis of androgens, while CYP19a1 encodes aromatase **(Fig. 2)**.[10]

■ DOSAGE

Berberine is generally well tolerated and is associated with few reported side effects. However, it may interact with certain medications, including those metabolized by the liver or antidiabetic medications that lower blood sugar levels.

The optimal dosage of berberine varies depending on the specific health condition being addressed. Generally, a dosage of 500–1,500 mg/day, divided into two or three doses, is considered effective. It is essential to choose high-quality, standardized berberine supplements from reputable brands to ensure purity and potency as the commercially available preparations may show wide variability.

■ HEALTH BENEFITS AND CLINICAL APPLICATIONS

Blood Sugar Control

Several clinical trials have demonstrated that berberine can effectively reduce fasting blood glucose levels and hemoglobin A_1c (HbA_1c) levels, making it a perfect natural alternative to conventional antidiabetic treatment

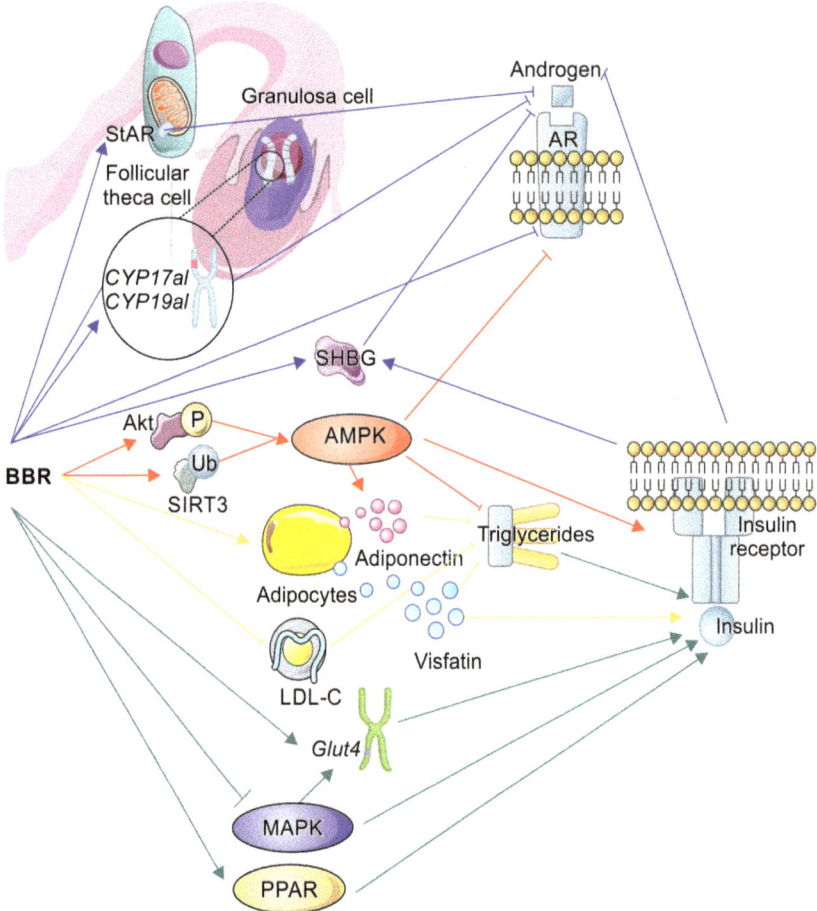

Fig. 2: Berberine (BBR) actions.[1] (AMPK: AMP-activated protein kinase; AR: androgen receptor; LDL-C: low-density lipoprotein cholesterol; MAPK: mitogen-activated protein kinase; PPAR: peroxisome proliferator activated receptor; SHBG: sex hormone-binding globulin; SIRT3: Sirtuin 3; StAR: steroidogenetic acute regulatory protein)

including insulin sensitizers like metformin. Hence, it has also shown promise in managing gestational diabetes, PCOS, and metabolic syndrome as well.

Cardiovascular Health

Berberine helps to lower LDL cholesterol levels and improves the lipid profile, which has beneficial implications for cardiovascular health. It has also exhibited anti-inflammatory and antioxidant properties, which amplify its benefits on cardiovascular function. Studies have demonstrated that supplementing with berberine may help reduce the risk of atherosclerosis and related cardiovascular health issues.

Gut Health

Berberine has antimicrobial properties, making it effective against a wide range of bacteria, viruses, fungi, and parasites. This is the reason why it was prescribed in ancient times in the first place.

It has been used in the treatment of various gastrointestinal infections, including *Helicobacter pylori*, a bacterium associated with gastric ulcers and stomach cancer. Furthermore, berberine's anti-inflammatory effects can help alleviate symptoms of inflammatory bowel disease, e.g., Crohn's disease and ulcerative colitis.

Weight Management

Research suggests that berberine may aid in weight loss, improve body fat distribution, and enhance body composition. It can accelerate fat breakdown, inhibit fat cell formation, and regulate appetite-regulating hormones, contributing to healthy weight management. Berberine's impact on metabolism and insulin sensitivity also plays a crucial role in these effects.

Anticancer Properties

Preliminary studies suggest that berberine exhibits anticancer properties by inhibiting the growth and spread of cancer cells. While more research is needed, berberine shows promise in combating various types of cancer, including breast, lung, liver, and prostate cancer. This is an exciting area of research, which holds much promise **(Fig. 3)**.

■ SCIENTIFIC EVIDENCE FOR COMBINATION THERAPY

Berberine and metformin can significantly increase the clinical pregnancy rate of PCOS patients, and berberine group also demonstrated a higher live birth rate. Berberine and metformin have similar effects on improving hyperandrogenism and hyperinsulinemia of PCOS patients, both of which can improve the pregnancy rate of PCOS patients undergoing IVF treatment and reduce the probability of OHSS.

Coadministration of berberine and metformin may not improve the effect of metformin on lowering body mass index (BMI) and HOMA-IR (Homeostatic Model Assessment for Insulin Resistance), but combining berberine with cyproterone acetate can improve glucose metabolism and insulin sensitivity, suggesting that berberine can be used as an insulin sensitizer.[11,12]

Berberine combined with drospirenone is an effective treatment for adolescent PCOS, which can significantly improve the sex hormone, glucose metabolism, and main clinical symptoms and signs in this condition.

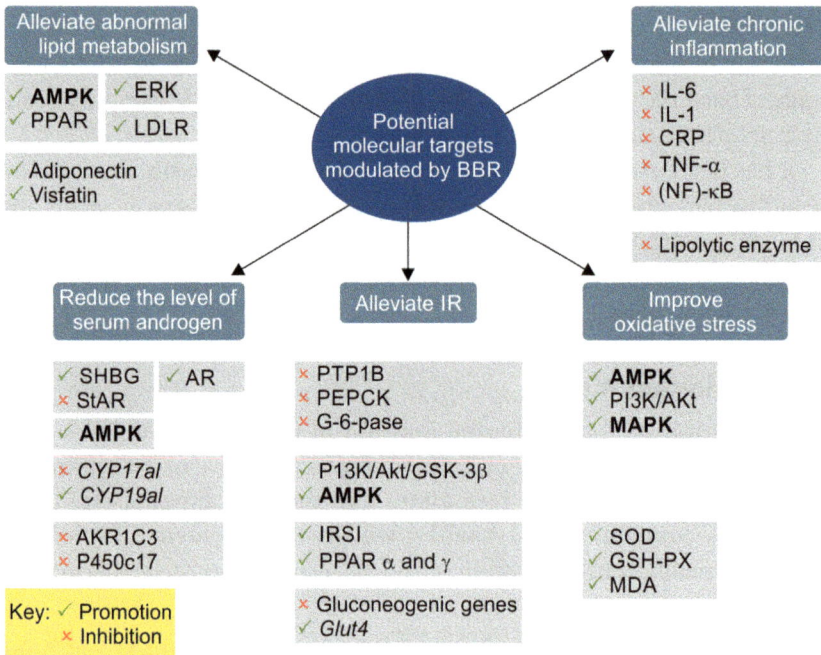

Fig. 3: Berberine targets for various actions.[1] (AKR1C3: aldo-keto reductase 1C3; AMPK: AMP-activated protein kinase; AR: androgen receptor; CRP: C-reactive protein; ERK: extracellular regulated kinase; G-6-pase: glucose-6-phosphatase; GSH-PX: glutathione peroxidase; IL-1: interleukin-1; IRS1: insulin receptor substrate-1; LDLR: low-density lipoprotein receptor; MAPK: mitogen-activated protein kinase; MDA: malondialdehyde; P450c17: p45017 α-hydroxylase; PEPCK: phosphoenolpyruvate carboxykinase; PPAR: peroxisome proliferator activated receptors; PTP1B: protein tyrosine phosphatase 1B; SHBG: sex hormone-binding globulin; SOD: superoxide dismutase; StAR: steroidogenetic acute regulatory protein; TNF-α: tumor necrosis factor alpha)

Berberine combined with letrozole has a synergistic effect on ovulation induction in PCOS patients with IR. The effect is better than metformin combined with letrozole and can significantly improve ovulation rates.[13]

Evidence from an Indian study has shown that berberine was associated with an improvement in various measures of IR that was comparable to that of metformin. The notable risk factors for metabolic syndrome and cardiovascular disease are increased waist circumference (WC), waist–hip ratio (WHR), and a deranged lipid profile. Berberine improved all these parameters and data suggest that berberine may have a greater potential to reduce cardiovascular disease risk than metformin in patients with PCOS **(Table 1)**.[14]

TABLE 1: Summary of clinical evidence.[1]

Combination drug	Patient(s)	Effect of experimental group compared with control group										
		BMI	HOMA (IR)	LH	T	FSH	LH/FSH	SHBG	FBG	FINS	Ovulation rate	Pregnancy rate
MET	56 women had PCOS	↓	↓	↓	↓	—	/	/	—	↓	↑	/
	Conclusion: Combining BBR with Met can improve the condition of BMI and IR more effectively as well as the rate of ovulation condition											
	84 obese women had PCOS	↓	↓	↓	—	↓	/	/	/	/	↑	/
	Conclusion: Combining BBR with Met can improve the obesity symptoms of obese women with PCOS, as well as reduce the hormone level and increase the ovulation rate											
CPA	100 women had PCOS	/	/	↓	↓	/	/	↑	/	/	/	/
	Conclusion: BBR intake improved some metabolic and hormonal disorders in a group of Chinese patients with polycystic ovary syndrome											
	80 infertile women had PCOS	/	/	↓	↓	↓	↓	↑	↓	↓	↑	/
	Conclusion: For patients with PCOS, CPA combined with BBR helps to regulate the fueling reproductive endocrine and glucose metabolism, promote the ovulation, increase pregnancy rate											
	50 women had PCOS	↓	↓	↓	—	/	/	/	↓	/	/	/
	Conclusion: BBR combined with CPA can effectively improve many pathophysiological changes, such as IR and high androgen levels in the treatment of PCOS											

Contd...

Contd...

Combination drug	Patient(s)	Effect of experimental group compared with control group										
		BMI	HOMA (IR)	LH	T	FSH	LH/FSH	SHBG	FBG	FINS	Ovulation rate	Pregnancy rate
Letrozole	644 women had PCOS	/	/	/	/	/	/	/	/	/	/	–
	Conclusion: For adolescents with PCOS, BBR combined with Yasmin can improve the endocrine metabolism and clinical symptoms significantly											
	98 PCOS patients with IR	/	/	/	/	/	/	/	/	/	←	/
	Conclusion: BBR combined with letrozole did not add fecundity in PCOS											
	Conclusion: BBR combined with letrozole can promote ovulation in PCOS patients with IR											
Clomiphene	120 infertile women had PCOS	/	↓	↓	↓	/	↓	/	/	→	←	←
	Conclusion: Combined BBR with clomiphene can improve endothelial function and endocrine, increase the rate of ovulation and pregnancy											

(BBR: berberine; BMI: body mass index; CPA: cyproterone acetate; FBG: fasting blood glucose; FINS: fasting insulin; FSH: follicle-stimulating hormone; HOMA (IR): Homeostatic Model Assessment for Insulin Resistance; LH: luteinizing hormone; MET: metformin; PCOS: polycystic ovary syndrome; SHBG: sex hormone-binding globulin; T: testosterone)

■ CONCLUSION

Berberine is a promising therapy, which has ancient roots in traditional medicine. It appears to have a wide range of health benefits. Through its multiple effects on blood sugar control, cardiovascular health, gut health, weight management, and cancer prevention, it has immense potential to form part of the modern clinician's armamentarium.

Alleviation of IR is the core mechanism of berberine in the treatment of PCOS. Other mechanisms can directly or indirectly affect IR. In addition, PPAR, MAPK, and AMPK signaling are the key pathways, which are affected. Due to the pharmacological effect of berberine, it is often used in combination with metformin, cyproterone, drospirenone, and other drugs in order to achieve better therapeutic results. Further research and large studies are necessary for its inclusion in everyday clinical practice.

■ REFERENCES

1. Zhang S, Zhou J, Gober HJ, Ting W, Leung WT, Wang L, et al. Effect and mechanism of berberine against polycystic ovary syndrome. Biomed Pharmacother. 2021;138:111468.
2. Wang Y, Fu X, Xu J, Wang Q, Kuang H. Systems pharmacology to investigate the interaction of berberine and other drugs in treating polycystic ovary syndrome. Sci Rep. 2016;6:28089
3. Chen C, Zhang Y, Huang C. Berberine inhibits PTP1B activity and mimics insulin action, Biochem Biophys. Res Commun. 2010;397(3):543-7.
4. Zhang N, Liu X, Zhuang L, Liu X, Zhao H, Shan Y, et al. Berberine decreases insulin resistance in a PCOS rats by improving GLUT4: dual regulation of the PI3K/AKT and MAPK pathways. Regul Toxicol Pharmacol. 2020;110:104544.
5. Yin TX, Wen J, Wei W, Li C. Effect of berberine on endometrial PPARs and endocrine metabolism of PCOS rat. Med Innov China. 2019;16(7):1-6.
6. Li W, Li D, Kuang H, Feng X, Ai W, Wang Y, et al. Berberine increases glucose uptake and intracellular ROS levels by promoting Sirtuin 3 ubiquitination. Biomed Pharmacother. 2020;121:109563.
7. Chen Y, Fu LL, Wen X, Wang XY, Liu J, Cheng Y, et al. Sirtuin-3 (SIRT3), a therapeutic target with oncogenic and tumor-suppressive function in cancer. Cell Death Dis. 2014;5(2):e1047.
8. Shen M, Zhang Z, Ratnam M, Dou QP. The interplay of AMP-activated protein kinase and androgen receptor in prostate cancer cells. J Cell Physiol. 2014;229(6):688-95.
9. Horman S, Vertommen D, Heath R, Neumann D, Mouton V, Woods A, et al. Insulin antagonizes ischemia-induced Thr172 phosphorylation of AMP-activated protein kinase alpha-subunits in heart via hierarchical phosphorylation of Ser485/491. J Biol Chem. 2006;281(9):5335-40.
10. Zhang Y, Zhao W, Han YH, Sun YH, et al. The effect of berberine on the treatment and curative effect of phlegm-damp PCOS rats. Chin Arch Tradit Chin Med. 2019;37(8):1807-12.

11. An Y, Zhang Y, Lu H, Li L, et al. Effect of berberine on clinical, metabolic and endocrine indexes and pregnancy outcome in women with polycystic ovary syndrome undergoing IVF treatment. Mod J Integr Tradit Chin West Med. 2016;25(5):459-62, 66.
12. Li MF, Zhou XM, Li XL. The effect of berberine on polycystic ovary syndrome patients with insulin resistance (PCOS-IR): a meta-analysis and systematic review. Evid Based Complement Altern Med. 2018:1-8.
13. Li HZ, Yu JF. Observation on the effect of berberine combined with letrozole on ovulation induction of polycystic ovary syndrome. J Pract Gynecol Endocrinol. 2016;3(10):84-6.
14. Mishra N, Verma R, Jadaun P. Study on the effect of berberine, myoinositol, and metformin in women with polycystic ovary syndrome: a prospective randomised study. Cureus. 2022;14(1):e21781.

CHAPTER 11

Astaxanthin

Parag Biniwale, Samidha Dalvi

■ BACKGROUND

Astaxanthin is a xanthophyll carotenoid which is found in various microorganisms and marine animals. It is a red fat-soluble pigment which does not have provitamin A activity in the human body, although some of the studies reported that astaxanthin has more potent biological activity than other carotenoids. The use of astaxanthin as a nutritional supplement has been rapidly growing in foods, feeds, nutraceuticals, and pharmaceuticals.

■ SOURCE OF ASTAXANTHIN

The natural sources of astaxanthin are algae, yeast, salmon, trout, krill, shrimp, and crayfish. Astaxanthin from various microorganism sources are presented in **Table 1**. The commercial astaxanthin is mainly from Phaffia yeast, *Haematococcus*, and through chemical synthesis. *Haematococcus pluvialis* is one of the best sources of natural astaxanthin **(Fig. 1)**.[1]

■ STRUCTURE OF ASTAXANTHIN

Astaxanthin is a member of the xanthophylls, because it contains not only carbon and hydrogen but also oxygen atoms **(Fig. 2)**. Astaxanthin has the molecular formula $C_{40}H_{52}O_4$. Its molar mass is 596.84 g/mol.

■ BIOCHEMISTRY OF ASTAXANTHIN[2]

Astaxanthin contains conjugated double bonds, hydroxyl, and keto groups. It has both lipophilic and hydrophilic properties. The red color is due to the conjugated double bonds at the center of the compound. This type of conjugated double bond acts as a strong antioxidant by donating the electrons and reacting with free radicals to convert them to be more stable product and terminate free radical chain reaction in a wide variety of living organisms.

TABLE 1: Microorganism sources of astaxanthin.

Sources	Astaxanthin (%) on the dry weight basis
Chlorophyceae	
Haematococcus pluvialis	3.8
Haematococcus pluvialis (K-0084)	3.8
Haematococcus pluvialis (Local isolation)	3.6
Haematococcus pluvialis (AQSE002)	3.4
Haematococcus pluvialis (K-0084)	2.7
Chlorococcum	0.2
Chlorella zofingiensis	0.001
Neochloris wimmeri	0.6
Ulvophyceae	
Enteromorpha intestinalis	0.02
Ulva lactuca	0.01
Florideophyceae	
Catenella repens	0.02
Alphaproteobacteria	
Agrobacterium aurantiacum	0.01
Paracoccus carotinifaciens (NITE SD 00017)	2.2
Tremellomycetes	
Xanthophyllomyces dendrorhous (JH)	0.5
Xanthophyllomyces dendrorhous (VKPM Y2476)	0.5
Labyrinthulomycetes	
Thraustochytrium sp. CHN-3 (FERM P-18556)	0.2
Malacostraca	
Pandalus borealis	0.12
Pandalus clarkia	0.015

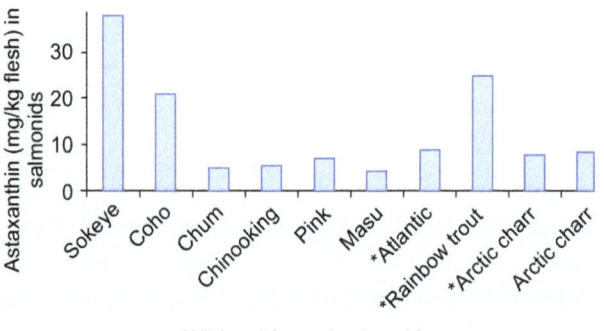

Fig. 1: Astaxanthin levels of wild and farmed salmonids.
*Salmonids

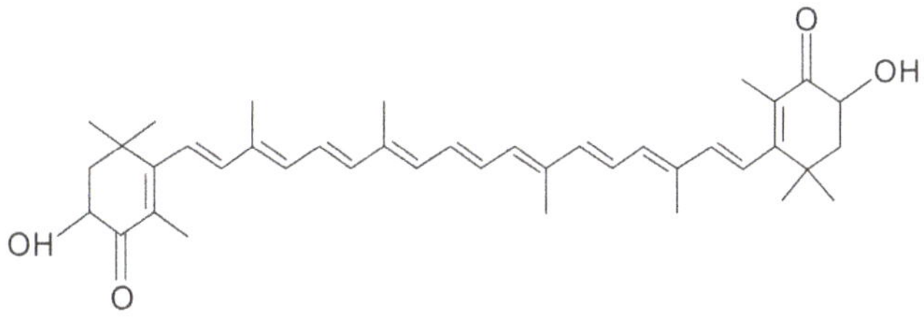

Fig. 2: Structure of astaxanthin.

BIOAVAILABILITY AND PHARMACOKINETICS OF ASTAXANTHIN

Bioavailability

Astaxanthin is a fat-soluble compound with increased absorption when consumed with dietary oils. Astaxanthin bioavailability in humans was enhanced by lipid-based formulations.

Pharmacokinetics

Carotenoids are absorbed into the body like lipids and transported via the lymphatic system into the liver. The absorption of carotenoids is dependent on the accompanying dietary components. A high cholesterol diet may increase carotenoid absorption while a low fat diet reduces its absorption. Astaxanthin mixes with bile acid after ingestion and make micelles in the intestinum tenue. The micelles with astaxanthin are partially absorbed by intestinal mucosal cells. Intestinal mucosal cells incorporate astaxanthin into chylomicra. Chylomicra with astaxanthin are digested by lipoprotein lipase after releasing into the lymph within the systemic circulation, and chylomicron remnants are rapidly removed by the liver and other tissues. Astaxanthin is assimilated with lipoproteins and transported into the tissues. Of several naturally occurring carotenoids, astaxanthin is considered one of the best carotenoids being able to protect cells, lipids, and membrane lipoproteins against oxidative damage.

BIOLOGICAL ACTIVITIES OF ASTAXANTHIN AND ITS HEALTH BENEFITS

- Antioxidant effects
- Antilipid peroxidation activity
- Anti-inflammation
- Antidiabetic activity
- Cardiovascular disease prevention
- Anticancer activity
- Immunomodulation

■ SAFETY AND DOSE OF ASTAXANTHIN

Astaxanthin is safe with no side effects when it is consumed with food. It is recommended to administer astaxanthin with omega-3-rich seed oils, such as chia, flaxseed, fish, nutella, walnuts, and almonds.[3] The combination of astaxanthin (4–8 mg) with foods, soft gels and capsules, and cream is available in the market. Recommended dose of astaxanthin is 2–4 mg/day.

■ ASTRAXANTHIN IN INFERTILITY

Astaxanthin and Male Infertility

Sperm Quality and Function

Several studies have demonstrated the positive effects of astaxanthin on sperm parameters including sperm count, motility, morphology, and DNA integrity. Notably, astaxanthin's antioxidant properties help neutralize oxidative stress, a major factor contributing to male infertility. Research studies by Zhang et al. (2016) and Fassett et al. (2018) reported significant improvements in sperm quality and function following astaxanthin supplementation.

Testosterone and Hormonal Balance

Astaxanthin has been shown to regulate hormonal balance in males including testosterone levels. Adequate testosterone levels are crucial for spermatogenesis and male fertility. A study by Comhaire et al. (2005) found that astaxanthin supplementation increased testosterone levels in infertile men, leading to enhanced sperm parameters and fertility outcomes.

However, in a randomized double-blind placebo controlled trial by Senka et al. in 2020, the authors concluded that the oral intake of 16 mg astaxanthin daily for 3 months did not significantly improve the semen parameters in patients with oligoasthenoteratozoospermia compared to placebo.

Astaxanthin and Female Infertility

Ovarian Function and Egg Quality

Astaxanthin exhibits protective effects against oxidative stress-induced damage in the ovaries. It has been reported to improve ovarian function, enhance oocyte quality, and regulate follicular development. Research by Mahmoud et al. (2019) and Li et al. (2020) demonstrated that astaxanthin supplementation in female infertility patients positively influenced ovarian reserve markers and increased the likelihood of successful pregnancy.

Astaxanthin in Polycystic Ovary Syndrome

Patients with polycystic ovary syndrome (PCOS) also suffer from endoplasmic reticulum (ER) stress. A randomized clinical trial by Masoome et al. (2023)

studied effect of astaxanthin treatment on ER stress in PCOS. The patients were classified into astaxanthin treatment (receiving 12 mg/day for 60 days) and placebo groups. A statistically significant increase was found in the follicular fluid level of total antioxidant capacity in the treatment group. Astaxanthin group had higher rates of high-quality oocytes, high-quality embryo, and oocyte maturity compared to the placebo group. The findings demonstrated that ER stress in the granulosa cells of PCOS patients could be modulated by astaxanthin.

Astaxanthin in Endometriosis

Oxidative stress and inflammation are interrelated and involved in the pathophysiology of endometriosis-associated infertility.[4] In a randomized, triple-blind, placebo-controlled clinical trial on 50 infertile endometriosis patients, the antioxidative, anti-inflammatory, and fertility-enhancing effects of astaxanthin supplementation were studied, which indicated that a 12-week supplementation with 6 mg/day of astaxanthin could effectively alleviate oxidative stress and inflammation and enhance assisted reproductive technology (ART) outcomes.

Endometrial Health and Implantation

Optimal endometrial health is essential for successful implantation and pregnancy. Astaxanthin's anti-inflammatory and antioxidant properties contribute to improved endometrial receptivity. Studies by Li et al. (2018) and Wang et al. (2021) found that astaxanthin enhanced endometrial thickness, reduced oxidative stress markers, and promoted favorable conditions for embryo implantation.

Mechanisms of Action

The beneficial effects of astaxanthin in male and female infertility can be attributed to its potent antioxidant and anti-inflammatory activities. Astaxanthin scavenges free radicals, protects against oxidative stress, reduces inflammation, and modulates gene expression related to reproductive function. These mechanisms collectively contribute to improved reproductive outcomes.[5]

Conclusion

The current scientific evidence suggests that astaxanthin supplementation holds promise as a therapeutic option for both male and female infertility. Astaxanthin's antioxidant and anti-inflammatory properties play a crucial role in improving sperm quality, hormonal balance, ovarian function, and endometrial health. While more research is warranted to establish optimal dosage, treatment duration, and potential interactions, astaxanthin offers a potential adjunctive therapy to conventional treatments for infertility. Further studies are necessary to validate its efficacy and safety in diverse patient populations.

ASTAXANTHIN IN OBSTETRICS

Astaxanthin inhibits H_2O_2-induced oxidative stress. Astaxanthin treatment significantly improved L-NAME-induced preeclamptic symptoms and reduced the oxidative stress and inflammatory damages in preeclamptic placentas. Astaxanthin treatment may effectively prevent and treat preeclampsia.

CONCLUSION

The current research data on astaxanthin is encouraging and have resulted from well-controlled trials in in vitro and in vivo models. Astaxanthin showed potential effects on various diseases including cancers, hypertension, diabetes, cardiovascular, gastrointestinal, liver, neurodegenerative, and skin diseases.

Its antioxidant properties are used against oxidative damage in diseased cells. Future research should focus on effects of astaxanthin esters on various biological activities and their uses in nutraceutical and pharmaceutical applications.

REFERENCES

1. Ambati RR, Phang SM, Ravi S, Aswathanarayana RG. Astaxanthin: sources, extraction, stability, biological activities and its commercial applications—a review. Mar Drugs. 2014;12(1):128-52.
2. Higuera-Ciapara I, Félix-Valenzuela L, Goycoolea FM. Astaxanthin: a review of its chemistry and applications. Crit Rev Food Sci Nutr. 2006;46(2):185-96.
3. Roche F. Astaxanthin As a Pigmenter in Salmon Feed, Color Additive Petition 7C02 1 1, United States Food and Drug Administration. Basel, Switzerland: Hoffman-La Roche Ltd.; 1987. p. 43.
4. Pashkow FJ, Watumull DG, Campbell CL. Astaxanthin: a novel potential treatment for oxidative stress and inflammation in cardiovascular disease. Am J Cardiol. 2008;101(10A):58D-68D.
5. Sarada R, Tripathi U, Ravishankar GA. Influence of stress on astaxanthin production in Haematococcus pluvialis grown under different culture conditions. Process Biochem. 2002;37:623-7.

CHAPTER 12: Levonorgestrel Intrauterine System

Krishnendu Gupta, Pratik Tambe

■ BACKGROUND

The levonorgestrel intrauterine system (LNG-IUS) is a device which has multiple uses in the field of gynecology. It is a small T-shaped device that is inserted into the uterus and releases a low dose of the hormone levonorgestrel. The LNG-IUS offers several benefits, including long-acting contraception, high effectiveness, a reduction in menstrual bleeding, and advantages of a one-time insertion leading to ease of use.

■ DEVICE CHARACTERISTICS

The LNG-IUS device is typically made of inert plastic, such as polyethylene. It is inserted into the uterus through the cervix by a healthcare professional during a quick and straightforward outpatient or office procedure, which does not require anesthesia. Once in place, the 52-mg LNG-IUS continuously releases a low dose of 20 µg levonorgestrel for a period of 7–8 years. After the recommended duration, the LNG-IUS can be removed or replaced **(Fig. 1)**.

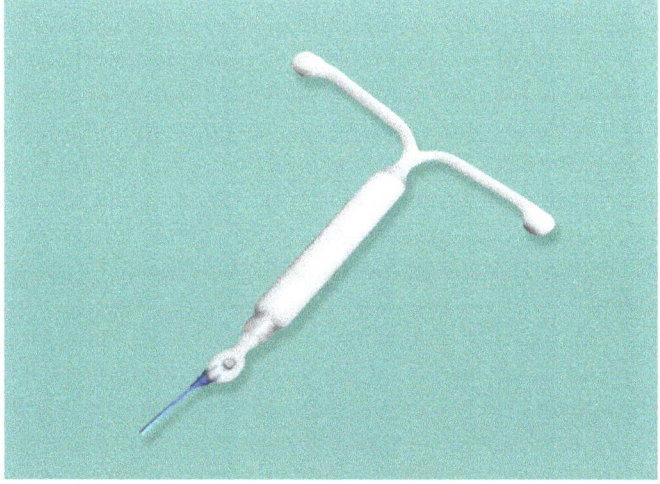

Fig. 1: Levonorgestrel intrauterine system.

■ MECHANISM OF ACTION

Levonorgestrel is a synthetic progestogen hormone similar to naturally occurring progesterone. Levonorgestrel released from the LNG-IUS primarily works by thickening the cervical mucus, hindering sperm movement, and prevents fertilization. It also thins the lining of the uterus, making it less receptive to implantation by a fertilized egg. This mechanism of suppressing the growth of the uterine lining leads to a reduction in menstrual bleeding.

■ DEVICE INSERTION

The insertion and removal of the LNG-IUS should be performed by a healthcare professional. The procedure is typically done in an outpatient setting and takes only a few minutes. Local anesthesia may be used to minimize discomfort during the insertion process. Removal of the LNG-IUS after the recommended duration is also a straightforward procedure.

■ CONTRACEPTIVE BENEFITS

One of the key advantages of the LNG-IUS is it is long acting in nature. With a duration of 7-8 years, the LNG-IUS offers hassle-free contraception without the need for a daily pill administration and/or frequent visits to healthcare providers. This results in reduced chances of contraceptive failure due to missed doses. Additionally, once inserted the LNG-IUS is invisible and does not interfere with daily activities, providing a discreet contraceptive option for women.

The LNG-IUS is generally a safe and suitable contraceptive option for most women. It can be used by women who have or have not given birth, women who are breastfeeding, and women who cannot use estrogen-containing contraceptives.

It is highly effective in preventing pregnancy. With a failure rate of <1%, it is considered one of the most reliable contraceptive methods available. It is more effective than oral contraceptive pills and comparable to other long-acting reversible contraceptives, such as implants and injections. The effectiveness of the LNG-IUS is not dependent on patient compliance and is not affected by other medications. However, it is important to note that the LNG-IUS does not protect against sexually transmitted infections (STIs), so additional measures such as barrier contraception should be considered for STI prevention.

Jensen et al., recently published their data of 362 patients; of which 243 entered and 223 completed 8 years of 52-mg levonorgestrel-releasing intrauterine system use. The mean (standard deviation) age was 29.2 (±2.9) years, and all participants were aged ≤36 years at the end of year 8. For years 6 to 8, the 3-year Pearl Index (95% confidence interval) was 0.28 (0.03–1.00) with a 3-year cumulative failure rate of 0.68% (0.17–2.71). Pearl Indexes for

TABLE 1: Pearl Index with LNG-IUS.[1]

Pearl Index during extended 52-mg LNG-IUS use up to 8 years

Pearl Index	Women (n)	Relevant exposure (WY)	Pregnancies (x)	Pearl Index, per 100 WY (95% CI)
3-year (years 6, 7, 8)	346	719.20	2	0.28 (0.03–1.00)
Year 6	362	296.87	1	0.34 (0.01–1.88)
Year 7	293	247.90	1	0.40 (0.01–2.25)
Year 8	229	194.42	0	0.00 (0.00–1.90)

Intention-to-treat analysis. Our mathematical model assumed that the number of pregnancies follows a Poisson-distribution.

Formula: PI = x/E; lower 95% confidence limit of PI = 0.5. $\chi^2_{(0.025, 2x)}$/E; upper 95% confidence limit of PI = 0.5. $\chi^2_{(0.075, 2(x+1))}$/E; where x = number of pregnancies, E = exposure in 100 WY (1 WY is 365 days of relevant exposure), $\chi^2_{(alpha, df)}$ is the alpha quantile from χ^2 distribution with df degrees of freedom.

(52-mg LNG-IUS: 52-mg levonorgestrel intrauterine system; CI: confidence interval; PI: Pearl Index; WY: women-years)

Source: Jensen et al.[1]

years 6, 7, and 8 were 0.34 (0.01–1.88), 0.40 (0.01–2.25), and 0.00 (0.00–1.90), respectively **(Table 1)**.

The discontinuation rate was 38.4% (139/362), most commonly because of desire for pregnancy (12.2%, 44/362). During extended use beyond 5 years, participants reported a decrease in the mean number of bleeding or spotting days with approximately half of the women experiencing amenorrhea or infrequent bleeding. At the end of year 8, most (98.7%, 220/223) of the participants who completed the study remained satisfied with the continued use of the 52-mg levonorgestrel-releasing intrauterine system. Of the 31 women who discontinued early because of desire for pregnancy, a 12-month return-to-fertility rate of 77.4% was reported.

They concluded that the 52-mg LNG-IUS maintains high contraceptive efficacy, user satisfaction, and a favorable safety profile through 8 years of use.[1]

■ UTILITY IN HEAVY MENSTRUAL BLEEDING

In addition to its contraceptive effectiveness, the LNG-IUS offers benefits for women's menstrual health. Many women experience a significant reduction in menstrual bleeding, with some even experiencing a complete absence of periods. This can greatly improve the quality of life for individuals who suffer from heavy or painful periods. Women using the LNG-IUS may also have fewer episodes of menstrual cramps or spotting between periods.

A Cochrane review published in 2020 of 13 randomized controlled trials (RCTs) included 3,174 patients from Egypt, Iran, China, Turkey,

Kuwait, Pakistan, and Norway. Treatment of endometrial hyperplasia with the LNG-IUS (1,657 patients) was compared with systemic progesterone (1,327 patients) or no treatment (190 patients). Systemic progesterone was administered orally in 12 studies and intramuscularly in one study. Endometrial hyperplasia was diagnosed through endometrial sampling (endometrial biopsy or suction curettage) with histologic evaluation. Sampling with histological examination was performed again at the end of the treatment period to determine treatment effectiveness.[2]

By the end of the treatment period, the LNG-IUS improved regression of endometrial hyperplasia compared with systemic progesterone or no treatment [at 6 months or less of treatment, odds ratio (OR) = 2.94; 95% CI 2.10–4.13; n = 1,108 and at 12 months of treatment, OR = 3.80; 95% CI 1.75–8.23; n = 138]. At 6 months or less of treatment, the rate of regression was 86% with the LNG-IUS and 72% with systemic progesterone. At 12 months, these rates were 80% with the LNG-IUS and 51% with systemic progesterone.

Treatment with the LNG-IUS was more effective overall at preventing hysterectomy than oral progesterone. In those treated with the LNG-IUS, the rate of hysterectomy was 11%, compared with 26% in those treated with oral progesterone (OR = 0.26; 95% CI 0.15–0.46; n = 452). The most common general adverse effects reported with both the LNG-IUS and systemic progesterone were spotting, nausea, and weight gain.

They concluded that there is moderate-certainty evidence for using the LNG-IUS for regression of endometrial hyperplasia versus systemic progesterone or no treatment. A dosage of 20 µg/day is reasonable for treating endometrial hyperplasia, but more research could help delineate the optimal dosage.

There is longstanding high certainty evidence for the many established benefits of the LNG-IUS, including decreased menorrhagia and fibroid volume regression, which, if untreated, could otherwise become nonmalignant reasons for hysterectomy. The LNG-IUS is an alternative to hysterectomy in management of endometrial intraepithelial neoplasia and endometrial hyperplasia for patients who wish to maintain fertility **(Table 2)**.

The American College of Obstetricians and Gynecologists also recognizes that the LNG-IUS for treatment of endometrial hyperplasia is an alternative to hysterectomy in appropriate patients.[3]

A more recent meta-analysis published 2022 included 341 studies, of which 12 were eligible. LNG-IUS yielded significantly higher resolution/regression rate (91.3% vs. 68.6%, OR 3.42, 95% CI 1.86–6.30). Failure and hysterectomy rates were significantly lower in LNG-IUS group compared to systemic progestins' group (19.2% vs. 32.3%, OR 0.34, 95% CI 0.20–0.57 and 9.3% vs. 24.1%, OR 0.41, 95% CI 0.29–0.57, respectively). They concluded that LNG-IUS is associated with high success rate in the management of women

TABLE 2: Forest plot levonorgestrel intrauterine system (LNG-IUS) versus nonuterine progestogens.

Study or subgroup	LNG-IUS Events	LNG-IUS Total	Oral progestogen/ No Rx Events	Oral progestogen/ No Rx Total	Weight	Odds ratio M-H, fixed, 95% CI	Odds ratio M-H, fixed, 95% CI	Risk of bias A B C D E F G
Short follow-up ≤6 months								
Abdelaziz 2013	31	42	24	42	14.9%	2.11 [0.84, 5.30]		
Abu Hashim 2013	40	59	29	61	21.7%	2.32 [1.11, 4.88]		
Behnamfar 2014	25	30	19	30	7.5%	2.89 [0.86, 9.74]		
Dolapcioglu 2013	51	52	50	52	2.3%	2.04 [0.18, 23.22]		
El Behery 2015	48	60	40	78	16.5%	3.80 [1.75, 8.23]		
Ismail 2013	30	30	58	60	1.5%	2.61 [0.12, 56.03]		
Karimi-Zarchi 2013	19	20	15	20	1.8%	6.33 [0.67, 60.16]		
Orbo 2014/2016	53	56	82	114	6.8%	6.89 [2.01, 23.65]		
Rezk 2016 (4)	47	54	86	108	17.6%	1.72 [0.68, 4.32]		
Rizvi 2018	65	70	56	70	9.5%	3.25 [1.10, 9.59]		
Subtotal (95% CI)		**473**		**635**	**100.0%**	**2.94 [2.10, 4.13]**		
Total events:	409		459					
Heterogeneity: $\chi^2 = 5.02$, df = 9 ($P = 0.83$); $I^2 = 0\%$								
Test for overall effect: $Z = 6.24$ ($P < 0.00001$)								
Long follow-up ≥ 1 year								
El Behery 2015	48	60	40	78	100.0%	3.80 [1.75, 8.23]		
Subtotal (95% CI)		**60**		**78**	**100.0%**	**3.80 [1.75, 8.23]**		
Total events:	48		40					
Heterogeneity: Not applicable								
Test for overall effect: $Z = 3.39$ ($P = 0.0007$)								
Test for subgroup differences: $\chi^2 = 0.35$, df = 1 ($P = 0.55$); $I^2 = 0\%$								

0.01 0.1 1 10 100
Favours oral progestogen   Favours LNG-IUS

with endometrial hyperplasia. However, specific effectiveness of LNG-IUS on more advanced histological subtypes is less studied.[4]

■ ENDOMETRIOSIS-ASSOCIATED PELVIC PAIN

A randomized controlled trial published 2018 comparing etonogestrel implant versus LNG-IUS demonstrated that both contraceptives improved significantly the mean visual analog scale endometriosis-associated pelvic pain and dysmenorrhea, without significant differences between treatment group profiles. Health-related quality of life improved significantly in all domains of the core and modular segments of the Endometriosis Health Profile-30 questionnaire, with no difference between both treatment groups. The most common bleeding patterns at 180 days of follow-up were amenorrhea and infrequent bleeding and infrequent bleeding and spotting among ENG implant and LNG-IUS users, respectively **(Table 3)**.[5]

A double-blind randomized controlled trial was conducted in 55 patients with endometriosis and moderate-to-severe dysmenorrhea (visual analog scale, greater than 50 mm) undergoing laparoscopic conservative surgery. After surgery, patients were randomized to a levonorgestrel-releasing intrauterine system ($n = 28$) or expectant management ($n = 27$) group. Compared with the control group, the LNG-IUS group had greater reduction in dysmenorrhea visual analog scale (−81.0 compared with −50.0 mm, $P = 0.006$) and pelvic pain visual analog scale (−48.5 compared with −22.0 mm, $P = 0.038$). The authors concluded that the LNG-IUS is effective and well accepted for long-term therapy after conservative surgery for patients with moderate to severe pain related to endometriosis. It can improve the patient's quality of life, including physical and mental health.[6]

■ SIDE EFFECTS

While the LNG-IUS offers numerous benefits, it may have potential side effects. The most common side effect reported is changes in menstrual bleeding patterns, e.g., irregular bleeding or spotting. Some women may experience lighter or shorter periods, while others may have heavier or longer periods initially. These changes usually settle over time, and many women find that their bleeding becomes lighter and more predictable.

Other potential side effects include headache, breast tenderness, nausea, acne, and mood swings. Most of these side effects tend to be minor and improve over time as the body adjusts to the hormone levels released by the LNG-IUS. It is important for patients to consult their healthcare provider if they experience any concerning or persistent side effects.

There are certain situations where the use of the LNG-IUS may not be recommended, such as in cases of active pelvic infection, certain types of congenital uterine abnormalities, or current or past history of certain

TABLE 3: ETN versus LNG-IUS for EAPP.[5]

EHP-30 results at baseline and at 180 days after device placement

Parameter	ENG implant			LNG-IUS		
	Baseline (mean ± SD)	180 days (mean ± SD)	P value	Baseline (mean ± SD)	180 days (mean ± SD)	P value
Core questionnaire:						
• Pain	68.7 ± 13.2	38.2 ± 19.3	<0.0001	65.2 ± 21.7	37.5 ± 17.7	<0.0001
• Lack of control or powerlessness	74.7 ± 16.3	42.2 ± 22.1	<0.0001	66.9 ± 23.6	35.9 ± 19.1	<0.0001
• Emotional well being	71.6 ± 18.1	46.9 ± 20.0	<0.0001	58.1 ± 21.3	43.1 ± 17.2	0.0007
• Social support	64.5 ± 23.9	42.9 ± 24.5	<0.0001	55.1 ± 24.6	44.5 ± 22.2	0.0284
• Self-image	62.8 ± 24.4	41.9 ± 23.2	<0.0001	50.3 ± 27.5	41.0 ± 26.2	0.0462
Modular questionnaire						
• Effect of endometriosis on:						
– Work	41.2 ± 30.5	21.3 ± 19.9	0.0002	38.8 ± 31.5	22.7 ± 20.3	0.0012
– Sexual intercourse	63.1 ± 29.9	38.9 ± 29.6	<0.0001	63.5 ± 29.7	42.5 ± 23.6	0.0004
– Relationship with children	28.8 ± 34.7	18.1 ± 21.8	0.0040	35.4 ± 34.6	21.8 ± 21.3	0.0061
• Feelings about the:						
– Medical profession	39.7 ± 29.8	26.6 ± 19.2	0.0082	43.1 ± 26.6	22.2 ± 14.7	<0.0001
– Treatment	55.0 ± 31.4	31.9 ± 17.5	<0.0001	53.8 ± 28.0	30.3 ± 15.1	<0.0001
– Possibility of not conceiving	51.2 ± 35.7	31.7 ± 30.3	<0.0001	36.7 ± 34.9	29.0 ± 28.8	0.0837

Source: Carvalho N et al.[5]
(EAPP: endometriosis associated pelvic pain; EHP-30: endometriosis health profile-30; ENG: etonogestrel implant; ETN: etonogestrel; LNG-IUS: levonorgestrel intrauterine system)

reproductive or uterine cancers. It is crucial to consult a healthcare provider to assess individual suitability and address any concerns or questions before considering the LNG-IUS as a contraceptive method.

Recently, there have been concerns regarding the theoretically higher breast cancer risk among LNG-IUS users. A meta-analysis published in 2021 did not find any increased risk in this population. Out of 494 studies, 294 studies were evaluated and 262 were excluded, because they did not meet the inclusion criteria. Out of 32 studies that were read in full, 24 were excluded. Thus, eight studies were included in the systematic review. The meta-analysis included four studies (two cohort and two case-control studies). Two subgroup analyses were performed for different study designs.

The estimated relative risk for the two cohort studies (144,996 cases), with moderate-quality evidence, was 0.93 (95% CI, 0.840-1.03). The odds ratio estimated for the two case-control studies (5,556 cases and 35,987 controls), with moderate-quality evidence, was 1.07 (95% CI, 0.91-1.26). Evidence of an increased risk of breast cancer was not observed in levonorgestrel-releasing intrauterine system users.[7]

■ CONCLUSION

In conclusion, the LNG-IUS offers a highly effective and convenient contraceptive option for women. With its long-acting nature, high effectiveness rate, reduction in menstrual bleeding, and ease of use, it provides a reliable and discreet contraceptive choice. It is also of immense benefit in women with heavy menstrual bleeding and endometriosis associated pelvic pain. While potential side effects exist, they are generally minor and improve over time. An increase in breast cancer risk among LNG-IUS users has not been found. As with any medical decision, it is important to consult healthcare providers to assess individual suitability and address any concerns before considering the LNG-IUS as a treatment modality.

■ REFERENCES

1. Jensen JT, Lukkari-Lax E, Schulze A, Wahdan Y, Serrani M, Kroll R. Contraceptive efficacy and safety of the 52-mg levonorgestrel intrauterine system for up to 8 years: findings from the Mirena Extension Trial. Am J Obstet Gynecol. 2022;227(6):873.e1-e12.
2. Mittermeier T, Farrant C, Wise MR. Levonorgestrel-releasing intrauterine system for endometrial hyperplasia. Cochrane Database Syst Rev. 2020(9):CD012658.
3. Silver S, Arnold JJ. Levonorgestrel-Releasing Intrauterine System for Regression of Endometrial Hyperplasia. Am Fam Physician. 2021;104(1):26-7.
4. Elassall GM, Sayed EG, Abdallah NA, El-Zohiry MM, Radwan AA, AlMahdy AM, et al. Levonorgestrel-releasing intrauterine system versus systemic progestins in management of endometrial hyperplasia: a systemic review and meta-analysis. J Gynecol Obstet Hum Reprod. 2022;51(8):102432.

5. Carvalho N, Margatho D, Cursino K, Benetti-Pinto CL, Bahamondes L. Control of endometriosis-associated pain with etonogestrel-releasing contraceptive implant and 52-mg levonorgestrel-releasing intrauterine system: randomized clinical trial. Fertil Steril. 2018;110(6):1129-36.
6. Tanmahasamut P, Rattanachaiyanont M, Angsuwathana S, Techatraisak K, Indhavivadhana S, Leerasiri P. Postoperative levonorgestrel-releasing intrauterine system for pelvic endometriosis-related pain: a randomized controlled trial. Obstet Gynecol. 2012;119(3):519-26.
7. Silva FR, Grande AJ, Lacerda Macedo AC, Colonetti T, Rocha MC, Rodrigues Uggioni ML, et al. Meta-analysis of breast cancer risk in levonorgestrel-releasing intrauterine system users. Clin Breast Cancer. 2021;21(6):497-508.

CHAPTER 13

Coenzyme Q10

N Sanjeeva Reddy, Radha Vembu

■ BACKGROUND

Infertility affects 15% of couples worldwide and one in six couples suffer from infertility.[1] In recent years, oxidative stress (OS) has been highlighted in the pathophysiology of infertility which is defined as the imbalance between the production of reactive oxygen species (ROS) and antioxidant defenses.[2]

■ FEMALE INFERTILITY

Aging leads to a continuous decline of the normal physiological process of ovulation. Oocyte quality is a critical prerequisite for fertilization and embryo development. With aging, there is a decline in de novo synthesis of coenzyme Q10 (CoQ10). So, supplementation of CoQ10 is advocated to improve the response to ovarian stimulation and improve the oocyte quality. Various interventions have been tried to improve oocyte quality. CoQ10 has gained importance due to its role in mitochondrial bioenergy, antioxidation, antiaging, and immune system regulation.

Coenzyme Q10 is a lipid-soluble quinone, which acts as an antioxidant, prevents lipid peroxidation, DNA oxidation as well as a bioenergetic molecule, empowering the body's energy production cycle through adenosine triphosphate (ATP) synthesis.[3] Meat, fish, nuts, and some oils are good sources of CoQ10. In humans, CoQ10 is synthesized from tyrosine.

Biochemical Properties and Physiological Functions

Coenzyme Q10 is found in reduced form (ubiquinol) or oxidized form (ubiquinone) and radical form (semiquinone). It is one of the vital constituents of the inner mitochondrial membrane. It plays an important role in electron transport in the mitochondrial respiratory chain and oxidative phosphorylation and functions as a lipid-soluble antioxidant in cell membranes and lipoproteins.[4] It is involved in ATP production in aerobic respiration.

Coenzyme Q10 has been studied in the management of pathological dysfunctions, such as diabetes mellitus, cancer, Parkinson's disease,

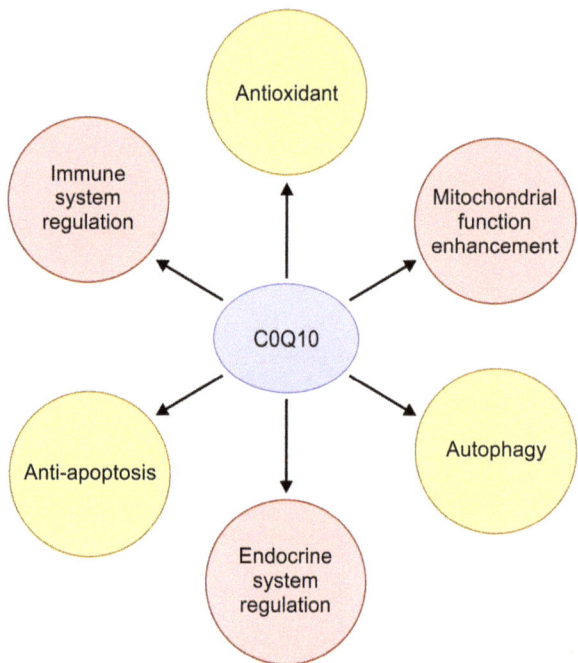

Fig. 1: Physiological functions of coenzyme Q10 (CoQ10).[6]

Huntington disease, heart disease, and infertility.[5] Its level is altered in pituitary diseases, such as acromegaly or secondary hypothyroidism **(Fig. 1)**.

Mechanism of Action

The role of CoQ10 to improve the oocyte quality and counteracting oocyte aging is studied. But the exact mechanism is not fully understood **(Fig. 2)**.

- *As a defense against oxidative stress*: Imbalance in production of ROS and OS can lead to DNA damage. This contributes to oocyte apoptosis which in turn leads to deterioration and degradation of regulation of oocyte maturation and fertilization.[8,9]
- *Effect of CoQ10 on ATP production and Krebs cycle*: Metabolites of Krebs cycle, i.e., citrate, malate, and fumarate, were reduced with aging and could be elevated back to levels seen in young controls with CoQ10 supplementation.[10]

Coenzyme Q10 and Aging

Reduced concentration of CoQ10 in plasma is associated with hypogonadism and altered levels of other steroid hormones.[11] It improves mitochondrial function, restores ROS imbalance, prevents DNA damage and oocyte apoptosis, and restores Krebs cycle downregulation from aging. There is

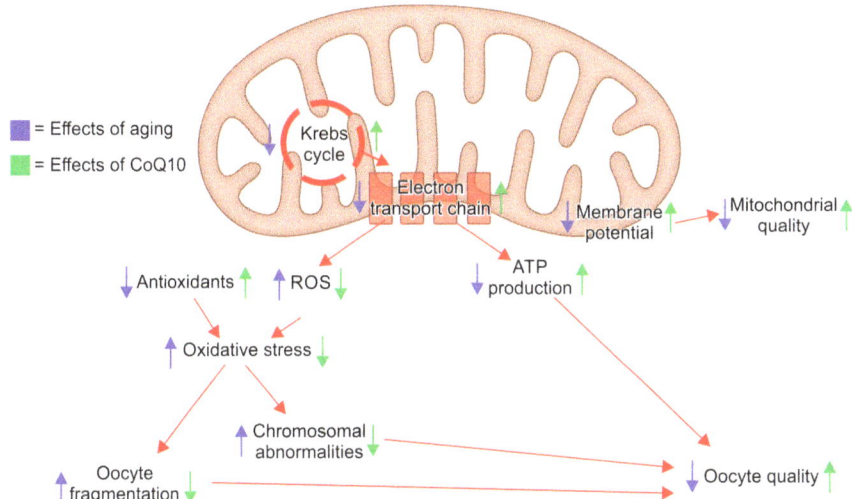

Fig. 2: Suggested mechanisms by which coenzyme Q10 (CoQ10) ameliorates the effects of oocyte aging;[7] purple arrows indicate effects of aging, while green arrows indicate effects of CoQ10. The direction of the arrow indicates whether the element is downregulated or upregulated. (ATP: adenosine triphosphate; ROS: reactive oxygen species)

age-related decline in CoQ10 levels more so in late 30s with increased rate of aneuploidy of embryos, suggesting a reduced expression of CoQ10 with ovarian aging.

In women >38 years, oocyte maturation was significantly higher when cultured with CoQ10 than in controls. There was reduction in postmeiotic aneuploidy rates. But in women <30 years, oocyte maturation, and aneuploidy rates were similar as in controls.[11]

Impact of Coenzyme Q10 on Ovarian Stimulation and Outcome

Clinically, supplementation of CoQ10 led to better response to ovarian stimulation and decreased odds of fetal aneuploidy in women with advanced maternal age. Pretreatment with CoQ10 resulted in significant decrease in the total amount of gonadotropin required for ovarian response, shorter duration of stimulation, higher peak estradiol levels, and number of oocytes retrieved.

Impact of Coenzyme Q10 on Oocyte and Embryo Quality[7]

- Coenzyme Q10 ameliorates effects of aging to improve chromosomal appearance, reduce chromosomal aneuploidy rates, and reduce fragmentation rates.

- It improves mitochondrial quality which can be implicated in oocyte quality and competency.

Coenzyme Q10 treatment also led to significantly more fertilization rate and number of high-quality embryos. Cycle cancellation rates due to no response to stimulation were significantly lower and less number of cancelled embryo transfers secondary to failed embryo development. There were more number of cycles with cryopreserved embryos.

In humans, CoQ10 is present in follicular fluid and its levels are significantly higher in mature oocytes when compared to dysmorphic oocytes. Similarly, levels were higher in grade I and II embryos than in grade III and IV embryos. It is shown that oral supplementation with CoQ10 increased the follicular fluid content and positively correlated with oocyte quality.[13]

The clinical pregnancy rates and live birth rates were higher following CoQ10 treatment even though it did not reach statistical significance.[14]

Coenzyme Q10 in a dose of 180 mg has shown improved response to ovulation induction with clomiphene citrate (CC) in CC-resistant women and has resulted in higher clinical pregnancy rate.[15]

There is paucity of knowledge of the role of CoQ10 on ovarian reserve even though beneficial effects are seen in rodents. The optimum dose and duration of administration of CoQ10 is still not very clear. It is used in a dose of 100–600 mg/day. But studies have shown that CoQ10 is well tolerated and safe for healthy adults at intake of up to 900 mg/day.[16]

Coenzyme Q10 in Polycystic Ovary Syndrome

Polycystic ovary syndrome (PCOS) accounts for 30% of cause for infertility among the infertile couples. The etiology of PCOS is not completely understood, although genetic and environmental factors have been attributed. At the cellular level, mitochondrial dysfunction, OS, and inflammation have been implicated in pathogenesis of PCOS.[17-19] Hence the rationale for investigating the therapeutic role of CoQ10 in the management of PCOS.

Coenzyme Q10 has been a safe therapy to improve PCOS by improving the insulin resistance. It increases the sex hormone levels, reduces testosterone levels, and improves the blood lipids.[20,21] CoQ10 is also shown to reduce the markers of inflammation [high-sensitivity C-reactive protein (hs-CRP), tumor necrosis factor alpha (TNF-α)] and endothelial dysfunction [vascular cell adhesion molecule (VCAM), intercellular adhesion molecule (ICAM), e-selectin] in overweight and obese PCOS women.[22]

■ MALE INFERTILITY

Approximately 50% of the causes of infertility are attributable to combined male and female factor and 25% is attributed to male factor alone. Among the male factor, >25% of cases are attributed as idiopathic cause.[23] OS and ROS are known to cause sperm DNA fragmentation (SDF) in 30–80% of cases.[24]

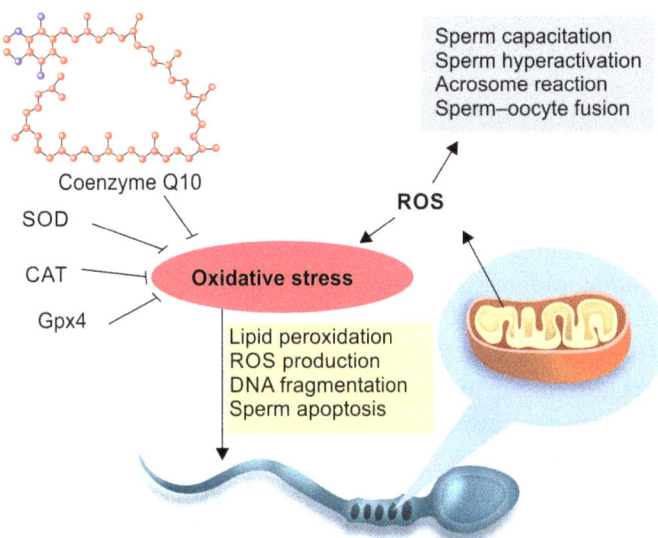

Fig. 3: Role of reactive oxygen species (ROS) and coenzyme Q10 on sperm function.[26] (CAT: catalase; Gpx4: glutathione peroxidase 4; SOD: superoxide dismutase)

Role of Oxidative Stress and Reactive Oxygen Species on Sperm Function

Small amounts of ROS are needed to ensure normal sperm cell functions such as capacitation, hyperactivation, acrosome reaction, and sperm–oocyte fusion, but excess ROS production induces OS. This can impair sperm membrane and DNA integrity leading to decreased sperm membrane fluidity, sperm motility, and changes in fertilizing capability of sperms **(Fig. 3)**.[25]

Mechanism of Action

Coenzyme Q10 acts as an antioxidant by inhibiting lipid peroxidation of the sperm membrane. The concentration of CoQ10 is more in the mitochondria-containing midpiece of the sperm which takes part in all energy-regulated processes.

Effect of Coenzyme Q10 on Semen Parameters

Supplementation of CoQ10:
- It increases the seminal CoQ10 levels.
- It improves the antioxidant capacity of seminal fluid.
- It improves both enzymatic and nonenzymatic germ cell production systems.

This protects sperm DNA from ROS damage and SDF improvement provides further evidence of usefulness of antioxidant therapy in male infertility.

Coenzyme Q10 supplementation has a positive effect on spermatogenesis. This is confirmed by reduction of follicle-stimulating hormone (FSH) and luteinizing hormone (LH) levels and increase in inhibin-B levels.

Supplementation of 600 mg/day of CoQ10 for 12 months in idiopathic oligoasthenoteratozoospermia patients showed significant increase in sperm concentration, progressive motility, and normal sperm morphology.[27] But a recent systematic review, CoQ10 monotherapy has shown a positive effect on seminal parameters. There was a significant increase in sperm concentration, but effect on sperm morphology is lower. But supplementation with compound mixes showed similar effects on sperm density, motility, and morphology.[26]

Deficiency of CoQ10 can lead to decreased sperm motility and sperm count. Studies have shown that supplementation of CoQ10 can improve the seminal fluid CoQ10 concentration which correlates positively with sperm motility, count, and morphology.

Effect of Coenzyme Q10 on Oxidative Stress Markers

Coenzyme Q10 is known to inhibit superoxide production, negative association is seen between CoQ10 and hydrogen peroxide. In men with idiopathic infertility, a significant increase in superoxide dismutase, total antioxidant capacity (TAC) glutathione peroxidase, and catalase activity is seen after CoQ10 treatment.[28,29]

Dose of Coenzyme Q10

Dose of CoQ10 varies from 20 to 600 mg/day in various studies. It has been used either as a monotherapy or along with other supplements vitamin C, vitamin E, carnitine, etc.

In a randomized controlled trial (RCT), 35 men with idiopathic oligoasthenoteratospermia (OAT) were treated for 3 months with CoQ10 at a dose of 200 mg/day and 30 patients with 400 mg/day. There was better improvement in semen parameters in men treated with 400 mg/day.[28] So overall, studies have shown that supplementation of CoQ10 raised seminal CoQ10 levels and improved the sperm parameters such as sperm concentration, and motility in male factor infertility. There is no consensus on the dosage to be prescribed.

Coenzyme Q10 and Sperm DNA Fragmentation

Among male factor, idiopathic infertility is the cause in 30% and SDF is one of the proposed mechanisms. DNA fragmentation can alter sperm function and decrease the chances of conception either naturally or by assisted reproductive technology (ART) conception. The increased OS can lead to DNA damage due to decreased protamination. CoQ10 present in human seminal fluid is involved in antioxidant, bioenergetics, and metabolic processes. Infertile men with high SDF levels showed a decrease in SDF after 3 months of antioxidant therapy including CoQ10.[30]

Effect of In Vitro Treatment of Gametes with CoQ10

Once the gametes are removed from their microenvironment, they can be exposed to excessive levels of ROS. So pretreatment with antioxidants might be beneficial to improve the quality of gametes. An in vitro study showed that incubation of spermatozoa for 3 hours with an antioxidant formula containing zinc, D-aspartic acid, and CoQ10 has shown beneficial effect on sperm motility, sperm recovery by swim-up technique and lipid peroxidation. So, this suggests that there is a place for these molecules prior to ART.[31]

■ CONCLUSION

- Coenzyme Q10 is naturally present in the body and is involved in the production of energy in the cells.
- Men with low CoQ10 have been associated with decreased sperm count, motility, and increased OS. Supplementation with CoQ10 may improve the markers of fertility.
- In females, supplementation of CoQ10 may improve fertility and more research is required to confirm these findings.
- Pretreatment with CoQ10 may improve the oocyte and embryo quality in young and old low prognosis patients with poor ovarian reserve.
- There may be possible beneficial effect on clinical pregnancy rate and live birth rate, but larger trials are required to confirm this.

■ REFERENCES

1. Farquhar C, Marjoribanks J. Assisted reproductive technology: an overview of Cochrane Reviews. Cochrane Database Syst Rev. 2018;8(8):CD010537.
2. Banerjee P, Bhattacharya J. Impact of oxidative stress on infertility, with emphasis on infertility management strategies. Glob J Fertil Res. 2019;4(1): 010-018.
3. Rodick TC, Seibels DR, Babu JR, Huggins KW, Ren G, Mathews ST. Potential role of coenzyme Q10 in health and disease conditions. Nutr Diet Suppl. 2018;10:1-11.
4. Vishvkarma R, Alahmar AT, Gupta G, Rajender S. Coenzyme Q10 effect on semen parameters: Profound or meagre? Andrologia. 2020;52:e13570.
5. Banihani SA. Effect of coenzyme Q10 supplementation on testosterone. Biomolecules. 2018;8:172.

6. Yang L, Wang H, Song S, Xu H, Chen Y, Tian S, et al. Systematic Understanding of Anti-Aging Effect of Coenzyme Q10 on Oocyte Through a Network Pharmacology Approach. Front. Endocrinol (Lausanne). 2022;13:813772.
7. Brown AM, McCarthy HE. The Effect of CoQ10 supplementation on ART treatment and oocyte quality in older women. Hum Fertil (Camb). 2023;1-9.
8. Mailloux RJ, McBride SL, Harper ME. Unearthing the secrets of mitochondrial ROS and glutathione in bioenergetics. Trends Biochem Sci. 2013;38(12):592-602.
9. Zhang M, ShiYang X, Zhang Y, Miao Y, Chen Y, Cui Z, et al. Coenzyme Q10 ameliorates the quality of postovulatory aged oocytes by suppressing DNA damage and apoptosis. Free Radic Biol Med. 2019;143:84-94.
10. Ben-Meir A, Burstein E, Borrego-Alvarez A, Chong J, Wong E, Yavorska T, et al. Coenzyme Q10 restores oocyte mitochondrial function and fertility during reproductive aging. Aging Cell. 2015;14(5):887-95.
11. Mancini A, Festa R, Raimondo S, Pontecorvi A, Littarru GP. Hormonal influence on coenzyme Q(10) levels in blood plasma. Int J Mol Sci. 2011;12:9216-25.
12. Ma L, Cai L, Hu M, Wang J, Xie J, Xing Y, et al. Coenzyme Q10 supplementation of human oocyte in vitro maturation reduces postmeiotic aneuploidies. Fertil Steril. 2020;114(2):331-7.
13. Turi A, Giannubilo SR, Brugè F, Principi F, Battistoni S, Santoni F, et al. Coenzyme Q10 content in follicular fluid and its relationship with oocyte fertilization and embryo grading. Arch Gynecol Obstet. 2012;285(4):1173-6.
14. Xu Y, Nisenblat V, Lu C, Li R, Qiao J, Zhen X, et al. Pretreatment with coenzyme Q10 improves ovarian response and embryo quality in low-prognosis young women with decreased ovarian reserve: a randomized controlled trial. Reprod Biol Endocrinol. 2018;16(1):29.
15. El Refaeey A, Selem A, Badawy A. Combined coenzyme Q10 and clomiphene citrate for ovulation induction in clomiphene-citrate-resistant polycystic ovary syndrome. Reprod Biomed Online. 2014;29:119-24.
16. Ikematsu H, Nakamura K, Harashima S, Fujii K, Fukutomi N. Safety assessment of coenzyme Q10 (Kaneka Q10) in healthy subjects: a double-blind, randomized, placebo-controlled trial. Regul Toxicol Pharmacol. 2006;44:212-8.
17. Zeng X, Huang Q, Long SL, Zhong Q, Mo Z. Mitochondrial dysfunction in Polycystic Ovary Syndrome. DNA Cell Biol. 2020;39:1401-9.
18. Mohammadi M. Oxidative stress and Polycystic Ovary Syndrome: a brief review. Int J Prev Med. 2019;10:86.
19. Dabravolski SA, Nikiforov NG, Eid AH, Nedosugova LV, Starodubova AV, Popkova TV, et al. Mitochondrial dysfunction and chronic inflammation in Polycystic Ovary Syndrome. Int J Mol Sci. 2021;22:3923.
20. Zhang T, He Q, Xiu H, Zhang Z, Liu Y, Chen Z, et al. Efficacy and safety of Coenzyme Q10 supplementation in the treatment of Polycystic Ovary Syndrome: a systematic review and meta-analysis. Reprod Sci. 2023;30(4):1033-48.
21. Izadi A, Ebrahimi S, Shirazi S, Taghizadeh S, Parizad M, Farzadi L, et al. Hormonal and metabolic effects of Coenzyme Q10 and/or Vitamin E in patients with Polycystic Ovary Syndrome. J Clin Endocrinol Metab. 2019;104:319-27.
22. Taghizadeh S, Izadi A, Shirazi S, Parizad M, Pourghassem Gargari B. The effect of coenzyme Q10 supplementation on inflammatory and endothelial dysfunction markers in overweight/obese polycystic ovary syndrome patients. Gynecol Endocrinol. 2021;37:26-30.

23. Punab M, Poolamets O, Paju P, Vihljajev V, Pomm K, Ladva R, et al. Causes of male infertility: a 9-year prospective monocentre study on 1737 patients with reduced total sperm counts. Hum Reprod. 2017;32:18-31.
24. Showell MG, Mackenzie-Proctor R, Brown J, Yazdani A, Stankiewicz MT, Hart RJ. Antioxidants for male subfertility. Cochrane Database Syst Rev. 2014;(12):CD007411.
25. Dutta S, Majzoub A, Agarwal A. Oxidative stress and sperm function: a systematic review on evaluation and management. Arab J Urol. 2019;17:87-97.
26. Salvio G, Cutini M, Ciarloni A, Giovannini L, Perrone M, Balercia G. Coenzyme Q10 and male infertility: a systematic review. Antioxidants (Basel). 2021;10:874.
27. Safarinejad MR. The effect of coenzyme Q_{10} supplementation on partner pregnancy rate in infertile men with idiopathic oligoasthenoteratozoospermia: an open-label prospective study. Int Urol Nephrol. 2012;44:689-700.
28. Alahmar AT, Sengupta P. Impact of coenzyme Q10 and selenium on seminal fluid parameters and antioxidant status in men with idiopathic infertility. Biol Trace Elem Res. 2021;199:1246-52.
29. Alahmar AT. The effects of oral antioxidants on the semen of men with idiopathic oligoasthenoteratozoospermia. Clin Exp Reprod Med. 2018;45:57-66.
30. Huang C, Cao X, Pang D, Li C, Luo Q, Zou Y, et al. Is male infertility associated with increased oxidative stress in seminal plasma? A-meta analysis. Oncotarget. 2018;9:24494-513.
31. Majzoub A, Agarwal A. Antioxidant therapy in idiopathic oligoasthenoteratozoospermia. Indian J Urol. 2017;33:207-14.

CHAPTER 14

Quatrefolate: The Fourth-Generation Folate

Ameya Purandare, Rohan Palshetkar, Manisha Nandi

■ BACKGROUND

Folate is an important vitamin for everyone required for all dividing cells including the production of red blood cells (RBCs). Folate is a substrate for an important reaction that involves a series of enzymatic reactions and cofactors, such as vitamin B_{12}, and it is necessary for the synthesis of DNA. Absorbed folates are metabolized in intestinal mucosal cells through a reduction and methylation to 5-methyltetrahydrofolate (5-MTHF) **(Fig. 1)**.

■ FOLIC ACID AND 5-METHYLTETRAHYDROFOLATE

Folate and folic acid must be converted to 5-MTHF before they can participate in the two key metabolic pathways: (1) methylation processes and (2) deoxyribonucleic acid (DNA) synthesis **(Fig. 2, Flowchart 1, and Fig. 3)**.

Quatrefolate passes the gastric barrier and is absorbed mainly in the small intestine by a carrier-mediated mechanism. The carrier is not saturated and this enables Quatrefolate to ensure a higher folate uptake.[1]

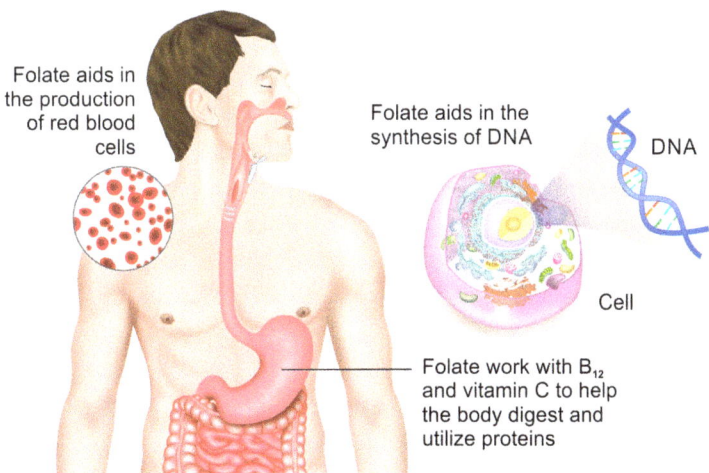

Fig. 1: Enzymatic reaction of folate. (DNA: deoxyribonucleic acid)

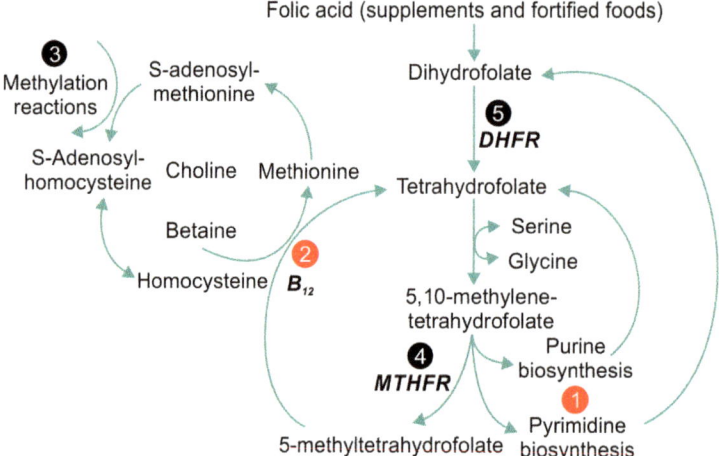

Fig. 2: Folic acid and 5-methyltetrahydrofolate process. (DHFR: dihydrofolate reductase; MTHFR: methylenetetrahydrofolate reductase)

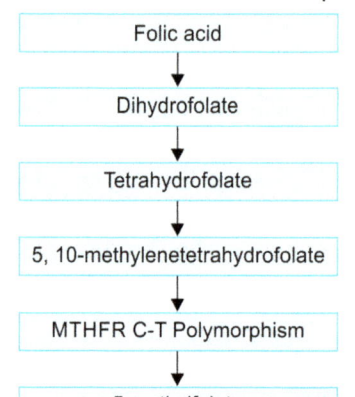

Flowchart 1: The conversion steps.

(MTHFR: methylenetetrahydrofolate reductase)

■ HEALTH BENEFITS OF THE DRUG

Humans need to maintain an adequate dietary intake of folate during various stages of their lives. Folate deficiency has far-reaching negative health consequences at all stages of life and has been implicated in the etiology of a variety of disorders including anemia, various forms of cardiovascular diseases, Alzheimer's disease, and osteoporosis, all of which have become pervasive health issues around the world in the 21st century **(Table 1)**.

The following are the uses of the drug:
- *Fertility:* The fourth-generation of folate bypasses the pathway of folate metabolism disturbances, improving fertility and increasing success rates

Quatrefolate: The Fourth-Generation Folate

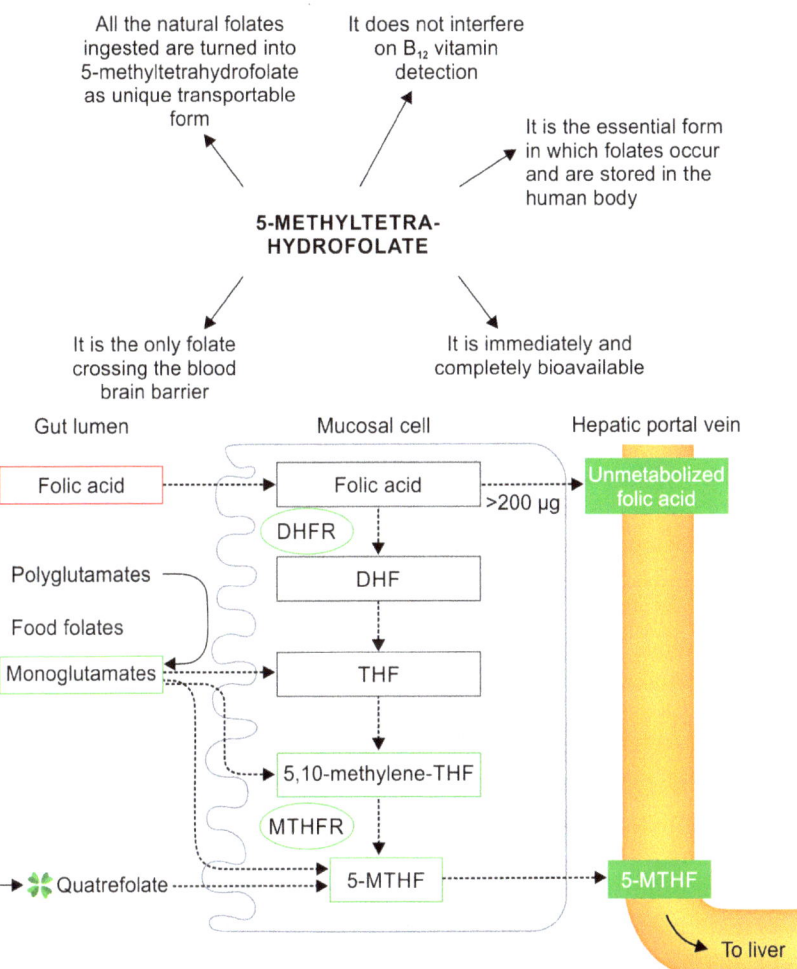

Fig. 3: Role of 5-methyltetrahydrofolate. (DHFR: dihydrofolate reductase; MTHFR: methylenetetrahydrofolate reductase; DHF: dihydrofolate; THF: tetrahydrofolate)

Table 1: Clinical researches emphasize the importance of folate supplementation.

- Neural-tube defect
- Male and female infertility
- Spontaneous abortion
- Coronary heart disease
- Macrocytic anemia
- Irritable bowel disease
- Cognitive deficits in elderly
- Lifestyle putting people at risk of low folate levels:
  - Smoking
  - Alcohol excess
  - eating disorders
  - Low vegetables intake
  - Chronic dieting
- Epilepsy
- Mood

in infertility treatment. Oxidative stress is one of the factors related to the pathogenesis of fertility disorders, such as idiopathic infertility, polycystic ovarian syndrome, and endometriosis. There was an inverse association between the frequency of multivitamin use with folate and ovulatory infertility.

- *Male infertility:* Folate levels measured in semen have been associated with sperm count and health. Low folate levels in semen were connected with poor sperm DNA stability.
- *Infants and children:* Folate is a critical nutrient when human cell growth is very active and folate deficiency can slow overall growth rate. Infants, children, and adolescents represent a critical phase of growth, and the proper level of folate is recommended to prevent a variety of medical conditions such as anemia.
- *Pregnancy:* During pregnancy, folate requirements increase to support embryonic and fetal development and maternal tissue growth, to reduce the risk of low birth weight, preterm birth, elevated homocysteine levels, and related adverse pregnancy outcomes. Maintaining sufficient levels of folate during pregnancy lowers the risk of neural tube defects (NTDs) and birth defects.
- *Spontaneous abortion:* Rapidly developing cells in the embryo may suffer from a lack of adequate folate. Failure to produce sufficient DNA and to regulate DNA function could lead to spontaneous abortion.
- *Down syndrome:* Several studies have investigated maternal enzyme polymorphism in the metabolization of folate as a risk factor for Down syndrome.
- *Lactation:* Breast milk folate concentrations are maintained at the expense of maternal folate reserves. A lactating woman would require 128 µg/day of additional folate in order to restore her losses. 5-MTHF appeared to be as effective as, and perhaps more effective than, folic acid in preserving RBC folate concentrations during lactation.
- *Menopause:* The drug is a safe and effective option for all women, helpful not only for hot flushes but for general women's health.
- *Cardiovascular:* The drug promotes healthier heart life reaching better blood levels of folate directly and translates to lower homocysteine levels, especially for patients with methylenetetrahydrofolate reductase (MTHFR) polymorphism.[2]
- *Glucose metabolism:* Lower folate levels are often observed in diabetic patients and result in high homocysteine levels, a recognized risk factor for cardiovascular disease and type 2 diabetes.
- *Cognitive and mood:* The active form of 5-MTHF is needed in the brain for the synthesis of norepinephrine, serotonin, and dopamine (**Flowchart 2 and Fig. 4**).[3]

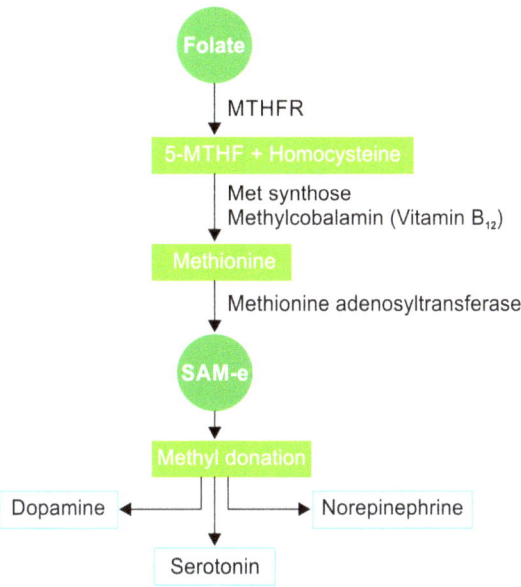

Flowchart 2: Synthesis of folate.

(MTHFR: methylenetetrahydrofolate reductase)

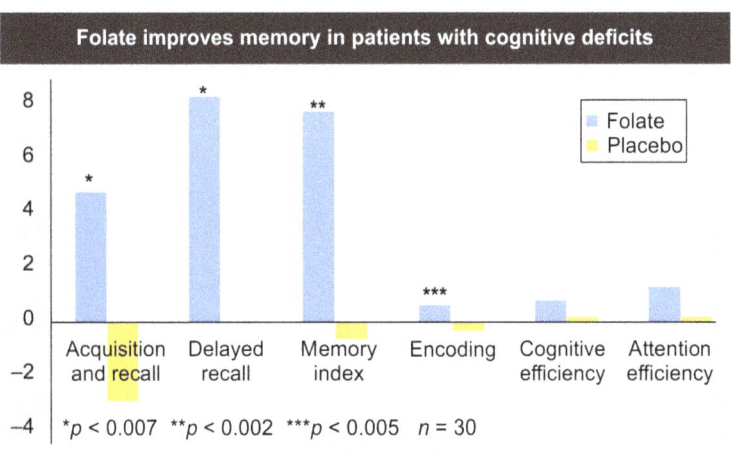

Fig. 4: Improvement in memory in patient with cognitive deficits.

In recent years, several studies have been published describing the biological pathways in which the reduced folate is involved. Folate is crucial for proper brain function and plays an important role in mental and emotional health.

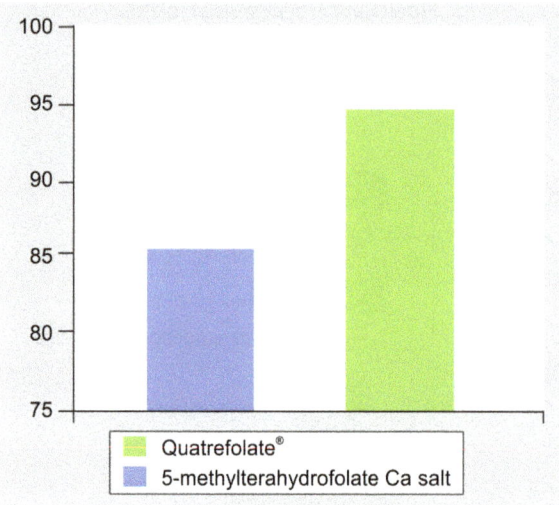

Fig. 5: Pharmacokinetic parameters for 5-methyltetrahydrofolate and Quatrefolate.

The innovative salt form overcomes the 5-MTHF calcium salt limits (the third generation) with significant advantages:
- *High water solubility:* High water solubility means the product may be better absorbed by mucosal cells which may facilitate access to the blood and circulation.
- *Improved bioavailability*
- *Long-lasting stability*
- *Established safety*

■ PHARMACOKINETICS

5-methyltetrahydrofolate bioavailability studies were performed in rats after po administration. The studies were performed also in healthy volunteers according to Good Laboratory Practice (GLP). The human clinical study confirmed the experimental findings in the rat: Quatrefolate has better bioavailability (+10%) than 5-MTHF.

Pharmacokinetic parameters (C_{max})-(6S)-5-MTHF calcium salt versus Quatrefolate (400 µg dose) **(Fig. 5)**.

■ CHEMICAL STABILITY (AT ROOM TEMPERATURE)

Besides the high chemical stability, the drug showed a very high solubility in water even higher than 1 g/mL compared with the slight water solubility of 5-MTHF calcium salt (1.1 g/100 mL) **(Table 2)**.

Table 2: Chemical stability of Quatrefolate.

Time 0		6 months		12 months		19 months	
Purity	Assay	Purity	Assay	Purity	Assay	Purity	Assay
99.3%	55.7%	99.0%	55.4%	98.5%	55.1%	98.3%	55.0%

■ TOXICOLOGICAL STUDIES

In Vitro

Bacterial Mutation in Salmonella Typhimurium and Escherichia Coli

The bacterial mutation assay was performed in order to assess the compound's ability to induce gene mutation in *S. typhimurium* and *E. coli*. The reverse mutation assay was run in bacterial strains already mutant at the locus whose phenotypic effects are easily detected, and since many chemicals can demonstrate mutagenic activity only after metabolism to some reactive forms, the test was performed in presence and in absence of a rat liver metabolic system (S9 microsomal fraction). The test concluded that the fourth generation of folate does not induce reverse mutation in *S. typhimurium* and *E. coli* at doses up to 5,000 µg/plate.

Mutation in L5178YTK Mouse Lymphoma Cells

The assay was done in order to confirm the inability of the new drug to induce mutation in L5178YK mouse lymphoma cells cultured after in vitro treatment, and in absence or presence of a rat liver microsomal system. The test concluded that the drug does not induce mutations at concentrations up to 5,000 µg/mL.

Chromosomal Aberrations in Chinese Hamster Ovary Cells In Vivo

The assay was made in order to demonstrate the inability of the drug to induce any chromosomal aberration in the presence or absence of a S9 liver microsomal fraction. No chromosomal aberrations were observed in Chinese hamster ovary (CHO) after in vitro treatment with the concentration of the drug up to 5,000 µg/mL.

In Vivo

Single Dose Oral Toxicity

The acute toxicity of the drug was assessed in rats of both sexes, dosing the product by gavage at 500 mg/kg level. After dosing, animals were observed for a 7-day period and finally sacrificed.

Established safety:

EU	When
Toxicological studies	Complete
GRAS report	July 2010
NDIN filing (USA)	November 2010
EFSA filing (EU)	Q3 2010

The fourth-generation folate is endowed with long-lasting stability, very high-water solubility, and better bioavailability than the commercially available methylated reduced folates.

RECENT UPDATES: THE ACTIVE FOLATE AND PREGNANCY OUTCOME VERSUS FOLIC ACID

A recently published case series study has evaluated the effect of 5-MTHF glucosamine salt in couples with recurrent miscarriages, lasting for at least 4 years. 5-MTHF glucosamine salt has been supplemented in a B vitamin complex and chelated zinc at a dosage of 800 µg/day, according to the 5-MTHF glucosamine salt requirements in healthy women.[4] The study conclusion highlights that the conventional use of large doses of folic acid (5 mg/day) has become obsolete. A physiological dose of 5-MTHFR glucosamine salt (800 µg) bypasses the MTHFR block and is suggested to be an effective treatment for couples with fertility problems. In the trial, the selected population showed a strong link between an impaired folate cycle, due to the presence of polymorphism of the enzyme MTHFR, and consecutively the capacity to achieve conception and carry a pregnancy to term. The women distribution of the C677T was wild type 38%, heterozygous 45%, and homozygous 17%, very close to what is generally observed in the UK. Most of the women had previously been treated unsuccessfully with high doses of folic acid (5 mg/day).[3,5]

There is now strong evidence indicating that MTHFR isoforms are detrimental to fertility in women and men; in all couples of the study, at least one of the partners was a carrier of the two main MTHFR isoforms. Of the 33 couples, 13 spontaneous pregnancies were observed, at the end of the treatment and the other 13 pregnancies were obtained after assisted reproductive technology (ART), with an overall ongoing pregnancy rate of 86.7%. The supplementation of 5-MTHF instead of folic acid appears to be an effective treatment for patients carrying the above mutations, where the physiological dose of 5-MTHF glucosamine salt (800 µg) bypasses the MTHFR block.

On the contrary, excess folic acid intake leads to unmetabolized folic acid (UMFA) syndrome in this peculiar population; UMFA syndrome may increase cancer risks and cause immune dysfunction. UMFA generated by high doses of folic acid may induce a pseudo-MTHFR syndrome via a

Table 3: Recommended dietary allowances for folate for children and adults.

Age (years)	Male and females (µg/day)	Pregnancy (µg/day)	Lactation (µg/day)
–	Floate	–	–
1–3	150	–	–
4–8	200	–	–
9–13	300	–	–
14–18	400	600	500
19+	400	600	500

mechanism of substrate inhibition, inducing a reversal of the cycle and a resulting increase in homocysteine.

CONCLUSION

Most countries have established recommended intakes of folate through folic acid supplements or fortified foods **(Table 3)**. External supplementation of folate may occur as folic acid, folinic acid, or 5-MTHF. Naturally occurring 5-MTHF has important advantages over synthetic folic acid. It is well absorbed even when gastrointestinal pH is altered and its bioavailability is not affected by metabolic defects. Using 5-MTHF instead of folic acid reduces the potential for masking hematological symptoms of vitamin B_{12} deficiency, reduces interactions with drugs that inhibit dihydrofolate reductase and overcomes metabolic defects caused by MTHFR polymorphism. Use of 5-MTHF also prevents the potential negative effects of unconverted folic acid in the peripheral circulation. Finished formulations with Quatrefolate are in the limelight of new clinical studies, providing even more evidence of the real advantages in terms of efficacy and safety of the drug.

REFERENCES

1. Scaglione F, Panzavolta G. Folate, folic acid and 5-methyltetrahydrofolate are not the same thing. Xenobiotica Fate Foreign Compd Biol Syst. 2014;44(5):480-8.
2. Nutraingredients-usa.com. (2021). Quatrefolic, the active form of folate that guarantees 100% of folate supplements' benefits. [online] Available from: https://www.nutraingredients-usa.com/News/Promotional-Features/Quatrefolic-The-Benefits-of-Active-Folate [Last accessed August, 2023].
3. Gnosisbylesaffre.com. (2020). Quatrefolic®, the active folate for fertility. [online] Available from: https://gnosisbylesaffre.com/blog/quatrefolic-science-up-new-issue-active-folate-on-fertility/ [Last accessed August, 2023].
4. Teodorescu C, Gherghiceanu F, Pituru S. New concepts in the treatment of infertility. Quatrefolic® versus folic acid. Ginecologia Ro. 2017;4(1):58-60.
5. Ns-Healthcare. Quatrefolic® The Active Folate and Pregnancy Outcome vs Folic Acid. [online] Available from: https://www.ns-healthcare.com/pressreleases/quatrefolic-the-active-folate-and-pregnancy-outcome-vs-folic-acid/ [Last accessed August, 2023].

CHAPTER 15

Gonadotropins in Prefilled Syringe Form

Seema Pandey, Pratik Tambe

■ BACKGROUND

Gonadotropins are biological compounds that play a crucial role in the hormonal control of bodily functions including reproductive processes. They are peptide hormones that are produced by the pituitary gland in the brain. Gonadotropins act on the gonads, which are the male testes and female ovaries, to regulate the production and release of sex hormones and the development of gametes (sperm and eggs).

Traditionally, gonadotropin therapy has involved the use of powdered formulations that require reconstitution before administration. However, advancements in medical technology have led to the development of prefilled syringe forms of gonadotropins. These prefilled syringes offer numerous benefits, including convenience, improved accuracy, and reduced risk of contamination.

■ PREFILLED SYRINGE CONCEPT

The invention of prefilled syringe with gonadotropins has paved the way to convenient medication of patients with remote facilities. A prefilled syringe is a disposable syringe that is supplied already loaded with the substance to be injected. The solution is supplied as a prefilled syringe already containing the liquid for injection. A prefilled syringe is a single dose of medication to which a needle has been fixed by the manufacturer.

Earlier metal or glass syringes were used but with time plastics and disposable syringes gained popularity in protecting the syringe. Previously, they were available as pens containing recombinant follicle-stimulating hormone (FSH) with a dial which allowed precise dosing from 37.5 IU up to 900 IU. These have been recently introduced in India for the highly purified gonadotropins, human menopausal gonadotropin (hMG) and FSH as well **(Fig. 1)**.

■ COMPARISON WITH TRADITIONAL FORMULATIONS

Patient Convenience and Compliance

One of the key advantages of using prefilled syringe forms of gonadotropins is convenience. Traditional powdered formulations often require several steps

Gonadotropins in Prefilled Syringe Form

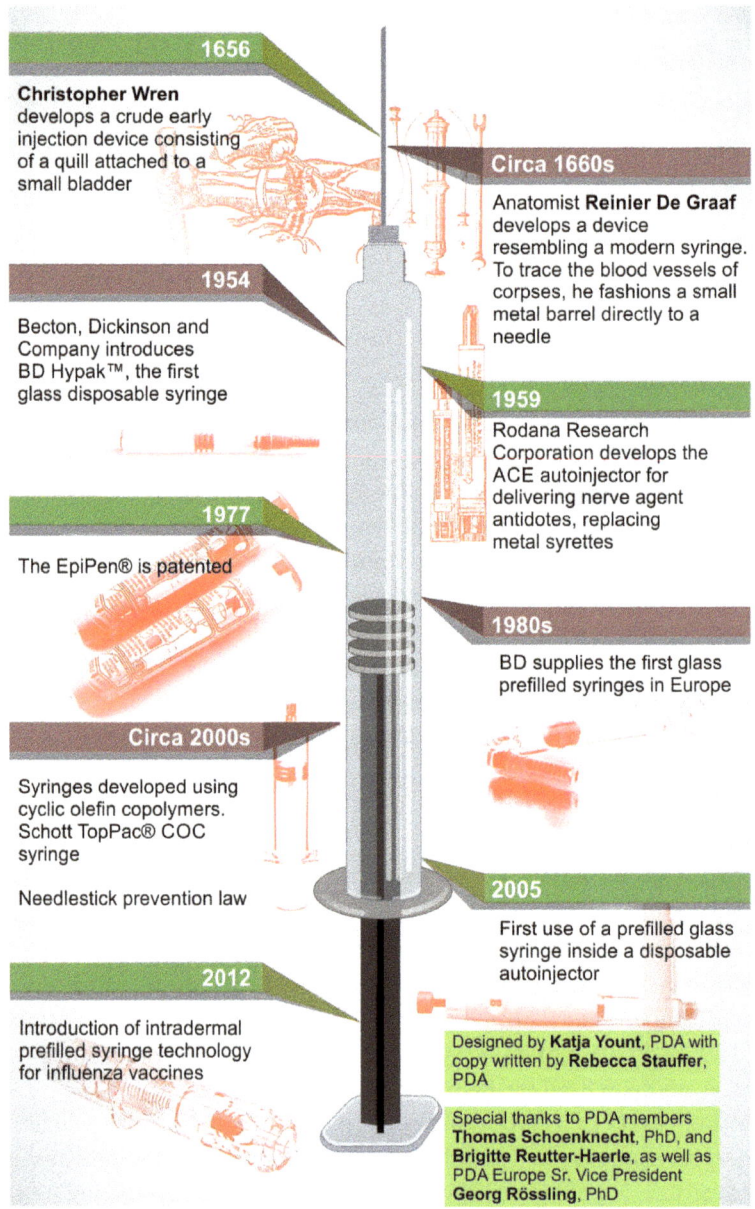

Fig. 1: History of prefilled medication syringes.

to reconstitute the medication before it can be administered. This process can be time-consuming and sometimes complicated, especially for patients who are self-administering the medication. Prefilled syringes eliminate the need for reconstitution, making the process of administering the medication simpler and more efficient.

The simplified administration process increases patient compliance and reduces the likelihood of errors in self-administration. The clear labeling on prefilled syringes provides easy to understand instructions, enhancing patient understanding, and minimizing the risk of mistakes.

Accurate Dosing

The accuracy of dosing is another significant advantage of prefilled syringe forms of gonadotropins. With traditional powdered formulations, there is a higher risk of measurement errors during reconstitution, which could result in under or overdosing. In contrast, prefilled syringes are precisely measured and labeled with the correct dosage, ensuring accurate administration and reducing the risk of adverse effects.

Less Painful

The integrated prefilled syringes have smaller gauge needles, e.g., 27G or 29G, which reduce pain and inflammation at the site of injection. This also makes them suitable for subcutaneous injection and self-administration **(Fig. 2)**.

Contamination Risk

Additionally, prefilled syringes help to reduce the risk of contamination. The sterile nature of prefilled syringes eliminates the need for handling the medication multiple times during reconstitution, reducing the likelihood of contaminating the drug with bacteria or other microorganisms. Additionally, prefilled syringes are sealed and tamper-proof, ensuring the integrity and safety of the medication.

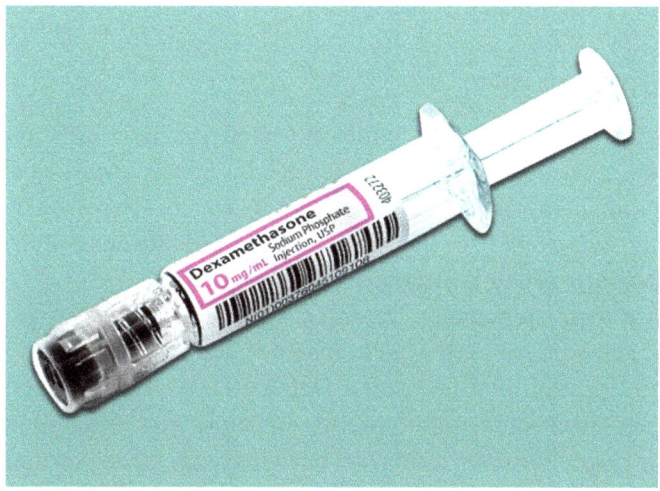

Fig. 2: Prefilled dexamethasone used in orthopedics.

Efficiency of Nursing Staff

In addition to these advantages, prefilled syringe forms of gonadotropins also offer practical benefits for healthcare providers. The ready-to-use nature of prefilled syringes eliminates the need for additional compounding steps, simplifying the overall administration process. This can save time for healthcare professionals, allowing them to focus more on patient care.

Positive Patient Experience

The ready-to-use nature of prefilled syringes makes them user-friendly, simplifying the medication administration process. This is particularly beneficial for healthcare providers who can focus on providing optimal patient care without the added complexity of reconstitution.

■ USAGE IN OTHER SPECIALTIES OF MEDICINE

Prefilled syringe medication delivery is already being practiced in other specialties, e.g., orthopedics and anesthesia where it has contributed to reduced errors in dosing, improved safety, clinician convenience, traceability, documentation, and accountability.[1]

■ SCIENTIFIC EVIDENCE

Prefills are useful for emergency situations and offer the possibility for duplicate peel-off labels, which aid in patient documentation. Preservatives are often not required for single-use prefilled syringes. According to a published review, 9 out of 10 healthcare professionals preferred prefills over conventional needles and syringes.[2]

■ DISADVANTAGES

It is important to note that while prefilled syringes offer numerous advantages, they may not be suitable or available for all patients or all types of gonadotropin therapies. Each patient's unique circumstances and treatment plan should be evaluated by their healthcare provider to determine the most appropriate form of administration.

Despite their advantages, prefilled syringe forms of gonadotropins may also have some limitations. For instance, they may be more expensive compared to traditional powdered formulations, as the manufacturing process and packaging requirements are more complex. Additionally, prefilled syringes may have a shorter shelf life compared to powdered forms due to stability concerns.

CONCLUSION

In conclusion, prefilled syringe forms of gonadotropins offer several benefits in the administration of hormonal therapies. They provide convenience, accurate dosing, reduced risk of contamination, and improved patient compliance. However, their use should be evaluated on an individual case basis to ensure compatibility with the patient's treatment plan and individual needs.

As medical technology continues to advance, it is likely that the development of prefilled syringe forms of gonadotropins will continue to evolve, further enhancing the delivery of reproductive health therapies. Supported by studies demonstrating their efficacy, prefilled syringes have revolutionized the fertility treatment and continue to play a crucial role in improving outcomes for patients undergoing assisted reproductive technology procedures.

REFERENCES

1. Kelly FE, Frerk C. Prefilled syringes have significant human factors benefits and would improve anaesthetic medication safety. Anaesthesia. 2023;78(7):921.
2. Makwana S, Basu B, Makasana Y, Dharamsi A. Prefilled syringes: an innovation in parenteral packaging. Int J Pharm Investig. 2011;1(4):200-6.

CHAPTER 16: Etonogestrel Implant

Basab Mukherjee, Riddhi Desai

■ BACKGROUND

As far as long-term contraception is concerned, women have multiple options and choices currently available to them. Etonogestrel implants are one of these and are widely used as a highly effective contraceptive option in women. These small, flexible rods are inserted under the skin and release a steady dose of the progestogen etonogestrel. Over the years, etonogestrel implants have gained popularity due to their long-acting nature, convenience, and reliability.

■ ETONOGESTREL

Etonogestrel is a synthetic progestogen that closely resembles the natural hormone progesterone **(Fig. 1)**. It has multiple modes of action, which enhance its efficacy as a contraceptive. Like other progestins, it works primarily by preventing ovulation, which is the release of an egg from the ovaries. By inhibiting ovulation, etonogestrel implants provide a highly effective contraceptive method. In addition, the hormone also thickens the cervical mucus, making it more difficult for sperm to reach the egg and alters the lining of the uterus, preventing the implantation of a fertilized egg.

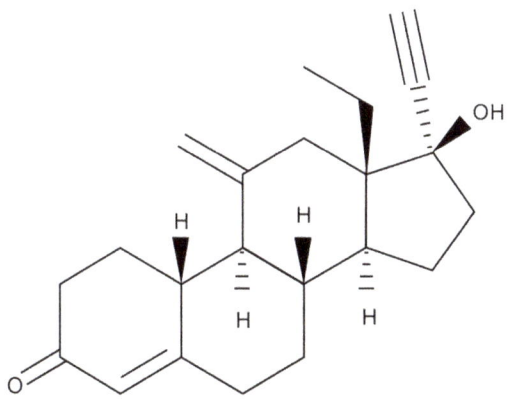

Fig. 1: Etonogestrel structure.

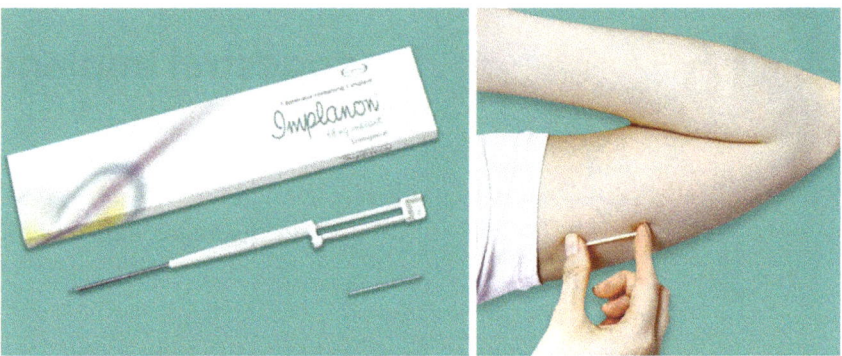

Fig. 2: Etonogestrel implant and placement site.

ETONOGESTREL IMPLANT

The implant itself consists of one or two small, flexible rods, typically about the size of a matchstick. The rods are inserted just underneath the skin of the upper arm by a healthcare professional during a quick and relatively painless procedure. Once in place, the etonogestrel implant releases a continuous low dose of hormone for a period of up to 3 years. After the 3-year period, the implant needs to be removed or replaced **(Fig. 2)**.

Compliance

One of the main benefits of etonogestrel implants is their long-acting nature. Currently, they are licensed for a 3-year duration, which ensures continuous contraception without the need for daily or frequent administration. This greatly reduces the chances of missing a dose and increases the user's compliance with the contraceptive method. Additionally, once the implant is inserted, it is invisible from the outside and does not interfere with daily activities, providing a discreet contraceptive option.

A 2-year-long study into contraceptive satisfaction and continuation rates among women in Malawi published in 2018 showed 96.3% continuation for etonogestrel implants. Immediate postpartum insertion of the device resulted in high patient satisfaction and is recommended to be offered routinely to eligible and interested women.[1]

Efficacy

Another advantage of etonogestrel implants is their high effectiveness rate. When used correctly, etonogestrel implants have a failure rate of <1%, making them one of the most reliable methods of contraception available. Compared to other long-acting reversible contraceptives, such as intrauterine devices (IUDs), etonogestrel implants offer a comparable level of effectiveness with less invasive insertion procedures.

Large studies have highlighted that the duration of effectiveness of the etonogestrel implant system is at least 2 years beyond the licensed duration of 3 years as recommended by the United States Food and Drug Administration (US FDA). A prospective cohort study started in 2012 and published in 2017 identified failure rate at the end of 4 years was 0 [97.5% confidence interval (CI) 0-1.48] per 100 woman-years. The failure rate at the end of 5 years was also 0 (97.5% CI 0-2.65) per 100 woman-years.[2]

The median etonogestrel level was 207.7 pg/mL (63.8-802.6 pg/mL) after 3 years. It was 166.1 pg/mL (67.9-470.5 pg/mL) after 4 years. It was still well maintained at 153.0 pg/mL (72.1-538.8 pg/mL) after 5 years. Median etonogestrel levels when compared to body mass index (BMI) showed overweight women having the highest serum levels (195.9, 25.0-450.5 pg/mL) when compared to normal weight women (178.9, 87.0-463.7 pg/mL) and obese women (137.9, 66.0-470.5 pg/mL) ($p = .04$).[3]

Menstrual Cycle Benefits

Additionally, etonogestrel implants have several benefits for users' menstrual cycles. Some women may experience a reduction in menstrual bleeding and cramping, leading to improved quality of life for those who suffer from heavy or painful periods. For others, menstrual bleeding may become irregular or even stop altogether. The contraceptive effect of the implant remains constant, regardless of changes in bleeding patterns.

Comparison with Levonorgestrel Implant

A study published in 2015 comparing the 3-year single-rod etonogestrel implant and the 5-year two-rod levonorgestrel (LNG) implants highlighted that both were associated with high patient satisfaction and continuation rates. The multicentric study took place in at multiple family planning clinics in several countries around the world, which included Brazil, Chile, Dominican Republic, Hungary, Thailand, Turkey, and Zimbabwe.

Etonogestrel and LNG releasing implants were found to be safe and highly efficacious in terms of contraceptive efficacy. The pregnancy rates were reported to be 0.0-0.5 per 100 women-years. The continuation rates for etonogestrel and LNG implants after 2.5 years were 69.8 (95% CI 66.8-72.6) and 71.8 per 100 woman-years (68.8-74.5), respectively.[4]

Side Effect Profile

Like any hormonal contraceptive, etonogestrel implants may have potential side effects. The most common side effects reported include changes in menstrual bleeding patterns, such as irregular bleeding or spotting. Some users may also experience headache, breast tenderness, mood changes, weight fluctuations, or acne. Most of these side effects tend to be minor and temporary, improving over time as the body adjusts to the hormone levels. However, it is important for individuals to consult their healthcare provider if they experience any concerning or persistent side effects.

Although etonogestrel implants are highly effective, it is important to note that they do not protect against sexually transmitted infections (STIs). Therefore, it is recommended to use additional barrier methods, such as condoms, to reduce the risk of STIs.

Breastfeeding

Etonogestrel implants are suitable for most women, including those who have not given birth, are breastfeeding, or cannot use estrogen-containing contraceptives. They are also a good option for women looking for long-term contraception without the hassle of daily pill administration.

A study published in 2018 from Malawi highlights that breastfeeding continuation was high at 21 months: 100% (95% CI 86.2-96.7) for etonogestrel implant users. 71% of etonogestrel implant users (95% CI 51.0-84.6) exclusively breastfed their infants until 6 months postpartum.[5]

Weight Gain Concerns

A study published from a University teaching hospital in Nigeria utilizing data over 7 years from 2007 to 2014 found that there was no statistically significant difference in weight gain among women belonging to different weight categories. Women with a preinsertion weight above 90 kg had weight gain <1 kg. Those who had <70 kg to begin with gained on average more than 2.0 kg. The most significant predictor of weight gain with etonorgestrel implant (ETN) implant use was the preinsertion body weight. This was able to predict weight gain 83.5% of the time (p value 0.000, CI 0.99-1.05).[6]

Contraindications

There are some instances when etonogestrel implants may not be recommended, such as in cases of known or suspected pregnancy, significant liver disease, or certain types of breast cancer. It is important to consult a healthcare provider to ensure that etonogestrel implants are the right choice for individual circumstances.

■ TRAINING AND EXPERTISE

The placement and removal of etonogestrel implants require the expertise of a healthcare professional. Insertion is typically a simple outpatient procedure performed under sterile conditions. The healthcare provider makes a small incision and inserts the implant just under the skin. Local anesthesia may be used to minimize any discomfort during the procedure **(Fig. 3)**.

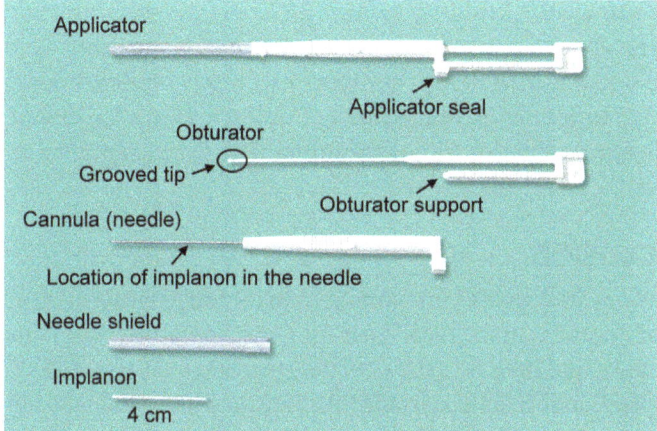

Fig. 3: Etonogestrel implant applicator.

Removal of the implant after the 3-year period is also a straightforward procedure. Removal takes approximately 50 seconds lesser time for the etonogestrel implant when compared to women who have the LNG implant ($p < 0.0001$) as per the 2015 study quoted earlier.[4]

The Family Planning Association of India (FPAI) and the Federation of Obstetric and Gynecological Societies of India (FOGSI) regularly conduct training programs for healthcare professionals, obstetricians, and gynecologists who wish to offer this to the patient populations that they cater to. The half-day training is comprehensive, with a standard program including presentations, videos, and hands-on training on mannequins and patients. At the end of the training, the candidate is presented with a training certificate testifying to their expertise and enabling them to offer ETN implants to their patients. The FOGSI Family Welfare Committee and the Ministry of Health have also helped in propagating this method of contraception throughout the country.

■ COST-EFFECTIVENESS IN INDIA

The Ministry of Health conducted an economic evaluation in 2021 to assess the economic feasibility of introducing the ETN implant into the Indian public healthcare system. A Markov cohort was conceptualized and the primary outcome was incremental cost-utility ratio (ICUR).[7]

Multiple sources for model inputs were considered including country-level data analysis, government reports, an observational primary costing study, a systematic review, and targeted literature reviews. The impact of etonogestrel implant introduction on the annual Indian health budget was also analyzed.

The base-case ICUR was Rs 16,475/- per quality-adjusted life-year gained. This demonstrated that ETN would be extremely cost-effective. The willingness-to-pay threshold is currently Rs 137,945. Budget impact analysis showed that introduction of the implant would account for <1% of the total annual health budget of India, assuming that the acceptance rates were 0.2–4%.[7]

■ CONCLUSION

In conclusion, etonogestrel implants are a highly effective form of long-acting reversible contraception. With their long-acting nature, low maintenance requirements, and high efficacy rate, they provide a reliable and convenient contraceptive option for women. While they may have potential side effects, these are generally minor and temporary. It is important to consult healthcare providers to assess suitability and address any concerns or questions before considering etonogestrel implants as a contraceptive method.

■ REFERENCES

1. Tang JH, Lemani C, Nkambule J, Talama G, Banda C, Zgambo W, et al. Two-year contraceptive continuation rates among immediate postpartum implant users at a district hospital in Malawi: a prospective cohort study. Contraception. 2018;98(3):220-2.
2. Ali M, Bahamondes L, Bent Landoulsi S. Extended Effectiveness of the Etonogestrel-Releasing Contraceptive Implant and the 20 μg Levonorgestrel-Releasing Intrauterine System for 2 Years Beyond U.S. Food and Drug Administration Product Labeling. Glob Health Sci Pract. 2017;5(4):534-9.
3. McNicholas C, Swor E, Wan L, Peipert JF. Prolonged use of the etonogestrel implant and levonorgestrel intrauterine device: 2 years beyond Food and Drug Administration-approved duration. Am J Obstet Gynecol. 2017;216(6):586.e1-586.e6.
4. Bahamondes L, Brache V, Meirik O, Ali M, Habib N, Landoulsi S; WHO Study Group on Contraceptive Implants for Women. A 3-year multicentre randomized controlled trial of etonogestrel- and levonorgestrel-releasing contraceptive implants, with non-randomized matched copper-intrauterine device controls. Hum Reprod. 2015;30(11):2527-38.
5. Krashin JW, Lemani C, Nkambule J, Talama G, Chinula L, Flax VL, et al. A comparison of breastfeeding exclusivity and duration rates between immediate postpartum levonorgestrel versus etonogestrel implant users: a prospective cohort study. Breastfeed Med. 2019;14(1):69-76.
6. Pam VC, Musa J, Mutihir JT, Karshima JA, Anyaka CU, Sagay AS. Body weight changes in women using Implanon in Jos, Nigeria. Afr J Med Med Sci. 2014;43(Suppl):15-21.
7. Joshi B, Moray KV, Sachin O, Chaurasia H, Begum S. Cost Effectiveness of Introducing Etonogestrel Contraceptive Implant into India's Current Family Welfare Programme. Appl Health Econ Health Policy. 2021;19(2):267-77.

Index

Page numbers followed by *f* refer to figure, *fc* refer to flowchart, and *t* refer to table.

A

Acetate 50
Acetic acid 33
Acidic pH 38
Acne, management of moderate-to-severe 51
Adenosine triphosphate synthesis 91
Adolescent endometriosis 29
Advanced cardiovascular life support 61
Aerobic respiration 91
Agrobacterium aurantiacum 76
Aldo-keto reductase 70*f*
Alphaproteobacteria 76
Alzheimer's disease 102
Androgen
    levels 67
    receptor 68, 70
Anemia 58, 102, 104
Angiotensin-converting enzyme inhibitors 61
Antiandrogenic effects, advantage of 54
Anticancer
    activity 77
    properties 69
Antidiabetic activity 77
Anti-inflammatory effects 43
Antilipid peroxidation activity 77
Antimineralocorticoid effects 50
    advantage of 54
Antioxidant
    defenses 91
    formula containing zinc 97
    properties 68
Antioxidation 91
Anxiety 38
Apoptosis 23
Appetite-regulating hormones, regulate 69
Arterial thromboembolic 54
Assisted reproductive techniques 44
Assisted reproductive
    technology 14, 15, 79
    conception 97
    procedures 115
Astaxanthin 75, 76*f*, 77-80
    beneficial effects of 79
    bioavailability of 77
    biochemistry of 75
    biological activities of 77
    dose of 78
    microorganism sources of 76*t*
    pharmacokinetics of 77
    safety of 78
    source of 75
    structure of 75, 77*f*
    supplementation 79
Asthma, severe 60
Atherosclerosis, risk of 68
Atopic dermatitis 37
Azoospermic infertile men 44
Azoospermic patients displaying 44

B

Bacillota 33
Bacterial mutation 107
Bactericidal factors 36
Berberine 65, 66, 72
    anti-inflammatory effects 69
    chemical structure of 65*f*
    coadministration of 69
Berberis 65
    aristata 65
    vulgaris 65
Beta blockers, treatment with 61
Biermer's disease 58
Bifidobacterium infantis 37
Bile acid metabolism 66
Biphasic pills 52
Bleeding 53
    irregular 119
Blood
    loss, frequency of 4
    pressure 61
    sugar control 67
Body
    iron stores, replenishment of 58
    mass index 69, 72
Bone mineral density 30, 31*f*
Breast
    cancer risk, higher 88
    tenderness 119
Breastfeeding 120

C

Cancer
  related anemia 58
  types of 69
Carbetocin 1-5
  chemical structure of 2f
  use of 4
Carbon dioxide 33
Cardiovascular disease 70, 102
  prevention 77
  risk 70
Cardiovascular health 68
Carnitine 96
Carotenoids 77
Catalase 95
  activity 96
Catenella repens 76
Cell membranes 91
Cellular apoptosis 23
Cellular senescence 23
Cervical mucus 53
Chemical stability 106
Chinese hamster ovary 107
  cells in vivo 107
Chlorella zofingiensis 76
Chlormadinone acetate 50
Chlorococcum 76
Chlorophyceae 76
Cholesterol
  from bloodstream 66
  synthesis 66
Chromosomal aberrations 107
Chronic inflammation 58
Chronic kidney disease 57, 58
Clinical researches emphasize 103t
Clomiphene 72
Clostridium difficile 37
Co-cyprindiol 51
Coenzyme Q10 91, 94, 95f, 96
  and aging 92
  concentration of 95
  de novo synthesis of 91
  deficiency of 96
  dose of 96
  effect of 95, 96
  impact of 93
  mechanism of action 92, 95
  physiological functions of 92f
  role of 92
  sources of 91
  supplementation of 91, 96
  treatment 94
Cognitive and mood 104
Cognitive deficits 105f
Combined hormonal contraception 49
Combined oral contraceptive pill 49
Commensal microbiota 34
Concomitant gastrointestinal pathology 58
Contraception, used for regular 53
Contraceptive method 118, 122
Conversion steps 102fc
Coptis
  chinensis 65
  japonica 65
Coronary heart disease 103
C-reactive protein 70
  high-sensitivity 94
Cyproterone acetate 51, 72
Cytochrome C 23

D

D-aspartic acid 97
Dehydroepiandrosterone 21
  clinical evidence 24
  in fertility, role of 22
  mechanisms of action 22
  structure 21f
  treatment duration 24
Deoxyribonucleic acid 43, 101
  fragmentation 96
Depression 38
Desogestrel 50-53
Desynchronizing ovulation 53
Diabetes mellitus 91
Diarrhea
  acute infectious 37
  antibiotic-associated 37
Dienogest 29, 31f, 50
  chemical structure 29
  chemical structure of 29f
  dosage and efficacy 30
  mechanism of action 29
  side effects 30
Dihydrofolate 103
  reductase 102, 103
Dihydrotestosterone, active form 43
Diminished ovarian reserve 22
Dopamine 104
Down syndrome 104
Downregulate proinflammatory cytokines 9
Drospirenone 51
  containing oral contraceptives 51
  only pill 54
Dydrogesterone 13, 15, 18

E

Ecological niche 36
Eczema 60
Efficacy 118
Egg quality 78
Elevated estrogen content 35
Embryo quality 93
Emergency contraception 8
Emergency contraceptive 7, 10
Emotional health 105
Endometrial biopsy 84
Endometrial cancer 9
Endometrial cells 9
Endometrial health and implantation 79
Endometrial hyperplasia 84, 86
Endometrial sampling 84
Endometrial transformation 53
Endometriosis 79
Endometrium 53
Endothelial dysfunction 94
Enteromorpha intestinalis 76
Enzyme, activity of 66
Epidermal growth factor 7, 30
Erythropoiesis 57
Escherichia coli 37, 107
Estetrol 51
Estetrol drospirenone combination 52
Estradiol 7
Estrogen 50
    containing contraceptives 49
    receptor 66
        expression of 53
Ethanol 33
Ethinylestradiol 50-52
Ethynodiol diacetate 50
Etonogestrel 117, 119
    implant 117, 118, 118*f*, 122
        applicator 121*f*
        removal of 120
    norgestimate 50
    structure 117*f*
Exhibited anti-inflammatory 68
Extracellular matrix 22
Extracellular regulated kinase 70

F

Facultative heterofermentative group 33
Farnesoid X receptor 66
Fasting blood glucose 72
    levels, reduce 67
Fasting insulin 72
Fat-soluble compound 77

Ferric
    carboxymaltose 59
    gluconate 59
    hydroxide 58
Fertility 102
    female 42
    male 43
    rate, improving 38
Fertilized egg 117
Fibroids, management of 7, 8
Florideophyceae 76
Folate 101, 109*t*
    active 108
    supplementation 103*t*
    synthesis of 105*fc*
Folic acid 101, 102*f*, 104, 108, 109
    doses of 108
    unmetabolized 108
Folinic acid 109
Follicle-stimulating hormone 24, 44, 49, 72
    receptor 24
Follicular fluid 94
Folliculogenesis, androgen effects on 24*f*
Forest plot levonorgestrel intrauterine system 85*t*
Four-phasic pills 52
Fourth-generation folate 101, 108
Fourth-generation progesterone 51*f*
Frozen embryo transfer cycles 14

G

Gametes, development of 111
Ganzoni formula 60
Gastrointestinal symptoms 9
Gene expression 22
    profile 22
Genetic markers 26
Genital tract, female 34, 35
Gestational diabetes mellitus 38
Gestodene 50
Glass syringes 111
Glucose metabolism 69, 104
Glucose-6-phosphatase 70
Glutathione peroxidase 70, 95, 96
Gonadal steroids, supraphysiological levels of 14
Gonadotropin 111
    forms of 111
    therapy 111
Gonadotropin-releasing hormone 14, 43
    agonists 8
Gonane derivatives 50
Gram-positive aerotolerant 33

Great emphasis 1
Growth factor 24
Gut health 69
Gynecologists 18

H

Haematococcus pluvialis 76
Hasten glycogen deposition 35
Headache 119
Health benefits of drug 102
Heart failure 57
Heat-killed probiotics 34
Heavy menstrual bleeding 9
Helicobacter pylori 69
Hemoglobin 57, 58
  A1C levels 67
High-molecular-weight iron dextran 58
Hirsutism 51
Homocysteine 109
Hormonal balance 78
Hormonal contraceptive 119
Hormonal imbalances 41
Hormone, low dose of 118
Human chorionic gonadotropin 14
Human immunodeficiency virus 36
Hydrastis canadensis 65
Hydrogen peroxide 36
Hypersensitivity reactions 60
  severity of 60

I

Idiopathic oligoasthenoteratospermia 96
Imferon 58
Immunoglobulin A 36
In vitro 107
  fertilization 21
Infections 43
Infertile
  couples 47
  teratozoospermic 44
Infertility 41, 78
  causes of 94
  female 78, 91, 103
  male 78, 94, 103, 104
  treatment of 41, 104
Inflammation, markers of 94
Inflammatory bowel
  disease 58
  syndrome 58
Inflammatory conditions 57
Inhibit fat cell formation 69
Injection, site of 113

Insulin
  like growth factor 1 receptor 24f
  receptor 66
    substrate-1 66, 70
  resistance 66, 72
    assessment for 69
Intensive care unit 1
Intercellular adhesion molecule 94
Interleukin-1 70
Intestinal barrier enhancement, probiotic
    mechanisms of 36f
Intestinal epithelial cell 34, 36, 101
Intracytoplasmic sperm injection cycles 22
Intramuscular iron preparations 60
Intrauterine
  devices 118
  insemination cycles 15
Intravenous iron 58
  preparations 58
Iron
  dextran 60
  isomaltoside 59
  malabsorption syndromes 58
  oxyhydroxide 58
  polymaltose 60
  sorbitex 60
  sucrose 59
Iron deficiency
  anemia 57
    iron-refractory 58
  stages of 57, 57f
Irritable bowel
  disease 103
  syndrome 37
Isolating probiotic-derived
    biomolecules 34

K

Kexin type 9 66

L

Labor, third stage of 1
Labyrinthulomycetes 76
Lactation 104
Lactic acid 33, 36
  accumulation 36
Lactobacillales 33
Lactobacillus 33, 35, 36, 38
  acidophilus 33
  bulgaricus 37
  colonize 34
  crispatus 35

gasseri 35
iners 35
jensenii 35
predominant environment 37
salivarius 33
species 33-36
types 33
uses of 34
Letrozole 72
Leukocytospermia 44
Leuprolide acetate 31*f*
Levomefolate 51
Levonorgestrel 50-53
extended cycle 52
implant 119
mechanism of action 82
releasing intrauterine system 9
Levonorgestrel intrauterine system 81, 81*f*
contraceptive benefits 82
device
characteristics 81
insertion 82
side effects 86
Lipid profile 68
Lipid-soluble
antioxidant 91
quinone 91
Lipoproteins 91
Liver
abscess 38
tumors, benign 53
Local corticotropin-releasing hormone system 43
Low-density lipoprotein
cholesterol 68
clearance of 66
receptor 70
Low-molecular-weight iron dextran 59
Lupus erythematosus 61
Luteal phase support 14
Luteinizing hormone 14, 49, 72
suppression of 15
Lymphoid tissue, gut-associated 34

M

Macrocytic anemia 103
Malacostraca 76
Male oxidative stress infertility, category of 43
Malignancy 58
Malignant liver tumors 53
Malondialdehyde 70
Massive blood transfusion 1
Mastocytosis 61

Maternal deaths 1
Maternal mortality rate 1
Matrix metalloproteinases 30
Mean corpuscular volume 57
Medroxyprogesterone acetate 50
Melatonin 41, 43
actions 46*f*, 47*f*
administration 47
exerts antiproliferative 43
functions 43
mechanisms of 41
receptors 43
structure 41*f*
supplementation 44, 47
synthesis 42*f*
treatment, impact of 44
Memory, improvement in 105*f*
Menopause 104
Menorrhagia, management of 53
Menstrual bleeding
patterns 119
utility in heavy 83
Menstrual cycle benefits 119
Mental health 105
Mestranol 50
Meta-analysis, largest 25
Metabolic syndrome 70
Metabolize contraception 54
Metal syringes 111
Metformin 70, 72
effect of 69
Methylation 101
Methylenetetrahydrofolate reductase 102, 103, 105
polymorphism 104
Methyltetrahydrofolate 101, 102*f*
phharmacokinetic parameters for 106*f*
role of 103*f*
Metronidazole 37
Miscarriage, threatened 16
Mitochondria nicotinamide adenine dinucleotide 66
Mitochondrial bioenergy, role in 91
Mitochondrial deoxyribonucleic acid 23
Mitochondrial function 23
Mitochondrial membrane's permeability 23
Mitochondrial respiratory chain 91
Mitogen-activated protein kinase 68, 70
Modulator-associated endometrial changes 10
Monophasic pills 51
Mood changes 119
Mouse lymphoma cells 107
Mucosal layer 34

N

Natural hormone progesterone 117
Neochloris wimmeri 76
Nestorone 50
Neural tube defect 103
    risk of 104
New generation oral contraceptive pills 49, 52
Newer progesterone-only pill 53
Nomegestrol acetate 50
Nonenzymatic germ cell production systems 95
Nonethylated estranes 50
Nonobstructive azoospermia 44
Nonuterine progestogens 85t
Norelgestromine 50
Norepinephrine, synthesis of 104
Norethindrone 50–53
Norethynodrel 50
Norgestimate 50–52
Norgestrel 50, 51
Nursing staff, efficiency of 114

O

Obesity 43
Obligate homofermentative group 33
Oocyte 93
    maturation, steps for 22
    quality 46f
Optimal endometrial health 79
Oral contraceptive pill 49
Oral dydrogesterone 15
Oral iron
    supplementation 57
    therapy 57, 58
        causes of in 58
        treatment failure in 58
Oral progesterone 84
Oral toxicity, single dose 107
Ormeloxifene 53
Osteoporosis 102
Ovarian follicle, melatonin action on 46f
Ovarian function 78
Ovarian hyperstimulation syndrome 14
Ovarian stimulation 25, 93
Oxidative phosphorylation 91
Oxidative stress 41, 43, 79, 91, 104
    damage 42
    markers 96
    role of 95
Oxytocin 5
    chemical structure of 2f
    continuous infusion of 4

P

Pandalus borealis 76
Pandalus clarkia 76
Paracoccus carotinifaciens 76
Parenteral iron 57
Parkinson's disease 91
Participant data meta-analysis 18
Pelvic pain, endometriosis-associated 29, 86
Peroxisome proliferator activated receptor 68, 70
Pharmacokinetic parameters 106
Phosphoenolpyruvate carboxykinase 70
Pill
    categories of 50
    ninety-one-day 52
Pineal gland 42f
    in brain 41
Pituitary downregulation 14
Pituitary gonadotropins, basal levels of 7
Polycystic ovary syndrome 66, 78, 94
Poor duodenal absorption 58
Poor ovarian reserve 21
Postgastrectomy 58
Postpartum hemorrhage 1
Postpartum iron deficiency anemia 58
Potent antioxidant 41
Prefilled dexamethasone 113f
Prefilled medication syringes, history of 112f
Prefilled syringe concept 111
Pregnancy 58, 104
    first trimester of 61
    hypertensive disorders of 1
    suspected 120
Probiotics
    safety of 38
    side effects of 38
    uses of 38
Progesterone 7
    only pills 52
    properties of 50
    receptor 7
Progestin-only pills 49
Progestogen 50
    etonogestrel 117
Proprotein convertase subtilisin 66
Protecting cells 41
Protein
    like cytochrome C 23
    tyrosine phosphatase 70
Pseudo-MTHFR syndrome 108
Psychological stress 43

Q

Quatrefolate 101, 106f
  chemical stability of 107t

R

Radical scavenger 43
Rat liver metabolic system 107
Reactive oxygen species 95
  production of 91
  role of 95f
Recurrent miscarriage 16
Red blood cells, production of 101
Reproductive endocrinologists 18
Reproductive health 38
Reproductive hormones, regulation of 41
Reticulocyte hemoglobin content 57
Rheumatoid arthritis 61
Room temperature 106

S

S9 microsomal fraction 107
Salmonella typhimurium 107
Salmonids 76, 76f
Scavenging harmful free radicals 41
Secretory immunoglobulin A 34, 36
Selective progesterone receptor
      modulator 7
Semen
  parameters 44, 95
  quality 43
Seminal CoQ10 levels 96
Seminal fluid 44
  CoQ10 concentration 96
Seminal plasma melatonin, levels of 44
Semi-systematic review 17
Senescent cells 23
Serotonin 104
Sertoli cells 44
Serum
  progesterone, levels of 17
  transferrin saturation 57
Sex hormone 69
  binding globulin 68, 70
  release of 111
Sexually transmitted infections 120
Sleep hormone 41
Sperm
  abnormalities 41
  concentration 43
  containing midpiece of 95
  deoxyribonucleic acid fragmentation 94, 96
  fertilizing capability of 95
  function 95, 95f
  membrane
    fluidity, decreased 95
    peroxidation of 95
  motility 43, 95, 96
    displaying impaired 44
  parameters 96
  quality and function 78
Spermatogonial stem cells proliferation 44
Spermatozoa, ejaculated 37
Spontaneous abortion 103, 104
Steroid hormone 13
Steroidogenetic acute regulatory
      protein 68, 70
Stimulate proton secretion 35
Suction curettage 84
Superoxide dismutase 70, 95, 96
Supplementing melatonin 42
Suprarenal cortex 21
Synthetic estrogen 50
Synthetic progestogen 117
  advantages of 50
Systemic inflammatory disease 61

T

Testicular function, restoring 43
Testis 43
Testosterone 78
  estranes derived from 50
Tetrahydrofolate 103
TFAM gene expression 23
Thraustochytrium sp. 76
Total antioxidant capacity 96
Traveler's diarrhea 37
Tremellomycetes 76
Trimegestone 50
Triphasic pills 52
Tumor necrosis factor
  alpha 70, 94
  gene 7
Tyndallized probiotics 35
Tyrosine 91
Tyrosine-protein phosphatase
      nonreceptor 66

U

Ulcerative colitis Crohn's disease 37
Ulipristal acetate 7, 10
  dosages advised 10
  side effects 9
Ulva lactuca 76
Ulvophyceae 76

Uterine bleeding, abnormal 8, 30
Uterus, lining of 117

V

Vaginal bacteria 35
Vaginal delivery 1
Vaginal epithelial cells 35
Vaginal epithelium 35
Vaginal flora, restoration of normal 38
Vaginal *Lactobacillus* 36
   protective benefits of 36
   species 37
Vaginal microbiome 37
Vaginal microflora diversity 38
Vaginal probiotic 36
Vaginal progesterone 15
Vancomycin 37
Varicocele 43
Vascular cell adhesion molecule 94
Venous thromboembolism 51
   risk of 49
Vitamin
   B_{12} deficiency, symptoms of 109
   C 96
   E 96

W

Water solubility, high 106
Weight gain concerns 120
Weight management 69

X

Xanthophyllomyces dendrorhous 76

www.ingramcontent.com/pod-product-compliance
Ingram Content Group UK Ltd.
Pitfield, Milton Keynes, MK11 3LW, UK
UKHW052202140425
457402UK00003B/19